The FODMAP Solution

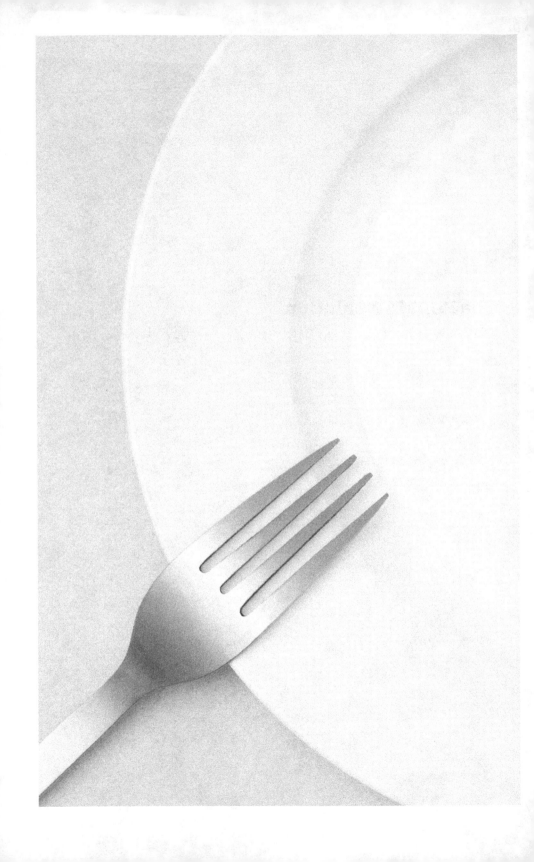

The FODMAP Solution

A Low-FODMAP Diet Plan and Cookbook to Manage IBS and Improve Digestion

SHASTA PRESS

For general information on our other products and services or to obtain technical support, please contact our Customer Care Department within the United States at (866) 744-2665, or outside the United States at (510) 253-0500.

Shasta Press publishes its books in a variety of electronic and print formats. Some content that appears in print may not be available in electronic books, and vice versa.

ISBN: Print 978-1-62315-350-2 | eBook 978-1-62315-351-9

Contents

Soups, Salads, and Sandwiches   69

Appetizers and Sides   87

Main Dishes   99

Desserts   123

Introduction

The word *diet* means different things to different people. In this book, diet is all about getting your body's digestive system back under control. If you are considering the low-FODMAP diet (FODMAP is an acronym for Fermentable Oligosaccharides, Disaccharides, Monosaccharides, And Polyols) for yourself or someone you know, then you already have a good idea of just how challenging life can be with a digestive disorder.

In Part One of the book, you'll be introduced to the low-FODMAP diet, which is an eating plan that helps you identify what foods work for you and what foods do not. The first step guides you in eliminating foods that can make you feel awful. The culprits have something in common—FODMAPs—which are thoroughly explained in the chapters that follow. Once your system has calmed down, the diet helps you discover your food tolerances and intolerances, so you know what you can eat comfortably, get back in control of your body, feel better, and stay healthy.

Once you have a clear idea of which foods are suitable for you, you'll want to put them together into a coherent eating program that is satisfying and nutritious. To make this task simpler, the book provides you with a 14-day menu plan to ease you into the diet. You can always substitute your own, favorite dishes, as long as the ingredients meet the FODMAP guidelines.

The advantage of a low-FODMAP eating plan is still coming into its own and research is still continuing. The Resources listed at the back of the book can help you stay on top of the latest developments and information.

In Part Two of the book, you will find a variety of tempting recipes for meals, snacks, appetizers, and desserts. Among them are modified or updated versions of traditional comfort foods, global favorites, and seasonal treats.

Read on, to discover the world of the low-FODMAP diet!

PART ONE

The Low-FODMAP Diet

In this part of the book, you will learn what FODMAPs are and the science behind your body's reaction to them. You will discover 10 common signs that you might have a digestive disorder and common treatments your doctor may prescribe. You will also learn more about foods that are low-FODMAP items so you can maximize them in your diet, as well as high-FODMAP foods to avoid during the preliminary phase of your diet. This book will also provide a section of answers to common questions about the low-FODMAP diet.

Moving from a basic understanding of a low-FODMAP diet to shopping at the supermarket, stocking your kitchen, or dining at your favorite restaurant may take some fine-tuning. A menu plan is provided for the acute beginning phase of the diet, when you will be limited to all low-FODMAP foods, as well as for the gradual and controlled reintroduction phase of some foods. The menu plan takes you from breakfast to dinner, with snacks, appetizers, and desserts, as well as offering strategies for dining out.

CHAPTER ONE

What Are FODMAPs?

We have learned that FODMAP stands for "Fermentable Oligosaccharides, Disaccharides, Monosaccharides, And Polyols." While you don't put saccharides and polyols on your grocery list or look for them on the menu, FODMAPs are in plenty of foods you eat, from such innocent seeming items such as fresh fruits and dairy to known unhealthful items like processed snacks and soft drinks.

FODMAP foods were first identified in 2001 by gastroenterologist Dr. Peter Gibson and nutritionist Dr. Sue Shepherd with their team at Monash University of Melbourne, Australia. What they found is that certain individuals with functional gastrointestinal disorders like irritable bowel syndrome (IBS) and a range of other digestive conditions are far less likely to suffer painful gastrointestinal symptoms and reactions when they limited ingestion of foods that are high in FODMAPs.

The foods that were the most likely to cause problems were high in lactose, fructose, fructans, galactans, and sugar alcohols (polyols), including:

- lactose: milk and milk products

- fructose: fruits, honey, and high-fructose corn syrup

- fructans: wheat, onions, and garlic

- galactans: beans, lentils, and soy

- polyols: stone fruits, avocados, and artificial sweeteners like sorbitol and manitol

The Science Behind FODMAPs

When you see the list of foods that are considered high-FODMAPs, you might wonder what they have in common. There are both "healthful" foods and "junk" foods in both high- and low-FODMAP groups. The answer is that they all contain carbohydrates.

Carbohydrates—simple and complex carbs and fiber—are concentrated in plant foods. Simple carbohydrates are listed on packaged food nutrition labels as sugars, which can be the sugars naturally found in milk, fruits, and vegetables or processed and refined sugars and syrups. Complex carbohydrates found in grains and legumes, as well as in fruits and vegetables, are sometimes referred to as starch. These carbohydrates are broken down in the gut by the bacteria that live there into the nutrients our bodies need. In addition, there are some carbohydrates that humans are not able to digest, known as fiber. Even though fiber doesn't supply nutrients to the body, it is still important to our health and digestive system. Soluble fibers have been shown to be part of keeping cholesterol levels and plaque low. Insoluble fiber has long been known for its ability to keep us "regular."

All these different types of carbohydrates share a characteristic: once they arrive in the gut, they begin to ferment. If something happens to disrupt the amount of bacteria at work in the gut or the amount of time a food spends in the gut, there can be several consequences.

Someone with a functional digestive disorder may be unable to digest certain carbohydrates for a variety of reasons. They may lack a specific enzyme or enough bacteria in the small intestine, for example. When carbohydrates aren't digested in the small intestine—a condition referred to as malabsorption—the bacteria in the large intestine suddenly find themselves with a bounty of the things they love to eat. The by-products of the bacterial feasting include acids, alcohols, and carbon dioxide, the same process that happens when yeast bread rises or beer is brewed. Since this is happening inside your gut, the gas is trapped. That's why some foods can make you not only feel but look bloated.

This is unpleasant enough, but it gets more complicated. Once fermentation is under way, it changes the pH of the gut, opening the door for a host of additional symptoms, ranging from gas to belching and inflammation to acid reflux. The rapid growth of the bacteria puts stress on the membranes lining the intestines and gut, and they become permeable. Important nutrients are able to leak out of the digestive tract before they are properly digested and absorbed.

In addition, these compounds are considered "osmotic" since they can attract and hold moisture. Bakers and pastry chefs take advantage of sugar's ability to attract and hold moisture to keep baked goods moist and flavorful for a long time. When someone sensitive to FODMAPs ingests sugar, they end up feeling, at the very least, bloated and uncomfortable.

The low-FODMAP diet has been around since 2001, but it has taken some time to gather evidence to support the benefits of the diet. Over time, though, increasing numbers of individuals have gotten relief from their IBS symptoms by cutting out high-FODMAP foods. Individuals with other conditions have also found it helpful.

10 Signs You Might Have a Digestive Disorder

If you haven't gotten a specific diagnosis for having a digestive disorder, you may still suspect that foods you are eating are making you sick. The reactions you have may be subtle, but you can still notice them. Eventually, you can even begin to anticipate them, since they happen every time you eat. There are a lot of reasons you might be suffering, from food allergies and celiac disease to lactose intolerance or even food-borne illnesses. Talking to your doctor and getting tested is critical.

Learning to avoid foods that are to blame and to concentrate on foods that don't make you suffer is the goal of the low-FODMAP diet. If the following symptoms describe you, this may be a sign that FODMAPs are to blame:

- Mealtime makes you vaguely anxious, because you know that in a few minutes or hours, you will start to feel cramps, or worse.

- You feel uncomfortable when you are out in public because you just can't tell when you will need to find a bathroom.

- Your stomach pains are so strong you cannot concentrate on work.

- Whether you get plenty of sleep or not, you feel worn out and exhausted.

- You have heartburn after you eat. Maybe over-the-counter antacids work or maybe you feel like you need something stronger.

- You don't plan outings in the great outdoors because there are no bathrooms.

- You are losing weight, and you are not trying to.

- You describe yourself as having a "sensitive" stomach.

- You turn down invitations because you really need to be close to your bathroom at home.

- Healthy foods like apples and onions make you feel uncomfortable, or worse.

- You can't remember the last time you felt like going to a restaurant; every time you go to one, you end up feeling sick.

There are several signs and symptoms of digestive disorders, some quite subtle and easy to overlook. People get used to the way they are and often just put up with it. When the symptoms get worse and worse, it only means that the condition has gone on untreated for longer and longer, doing more and more damage to your stomach and cheating your body out of the nourishment it needs.

Any digestive disorder is a serious condition. If you suspect that you have one, it is important to know exactly what kind of disorder you have. Pains that occur an hour or two after meals or in the morning, for instance, and go away after eating food or taking an antacid are typical of ulcers. IBS doesn't cause a skin reaction or wheezing, but a food allergy might. Your specific condition may be one that requires a medical treatment, possibly in combination with a low-FODMAP diet. Here are nine common signs of a digestive disorder to discuss with your doctor:

1. Persistent abdominal pain and cramps

2. Diarrhea

3. Fever

4. Blood in the stool

5. Bloating

6. Constipation

7. Weight loss

8. Gas

9. Persistent heartburn

Common Treatments Your Doctor May Prescribe

Before prescribing any treatment, including the low-FODMAP diet, your doctor will want to make sure you don't have some other serious intestinal condition with similar symptoms, including autoimmune diseases like celiac disease. Your doctor will need a detailed account of your condition, including when you experience symptoms, how frequently they occur, and whether anything specific causes a reaction or helps it to pass.

Beyond that, your doctor may suggest that you take different tests, such as blood tests, an upper or lower GI series, ultrasound, endoscopy, and barium GI studies. Some serious conditions may require a CAT scan or an MRI. It is possible that your doctor will take a biopsy during endoscopic procedures, since there could be other medical conditions involved. The FDA approved an effective breath test for peptic ulcers in 1996, for example, that makes diagnosis of this condition possible without an invasive procedure.

If you have a condition, your diagnosis may be one of the following:

- Inflammatory bowel disease (IBD)
- Crohn's disease
- Ulcerative colitis
- Diverticulitis
- Irritable bowel syndrome (IBS)
- Acid reflux (GERD)
- Peptic ulcer

Regarding digestive disorders such as Crohn's disease or IBS, doctors customize treatments and management programs to suit an individual's specific condition and its severity. The basic lifestyle modifications are the same ones you hear for most serious medical conditions:

- Stop smoking.
- Limit or reduce alcohol consumption and caffeinated beverages.
- Eat small meals.
- Get regular exercise and fresh air.
- Use meditation or relaxation techniques.

Different medications are available over the counter to treat conditions like heartburn, constipation, or diarrhea. When these symptoms are severe, your doctor can prescribe medications to deal with the symptoms. Options can include fiber supplements, antispasmodics, antacids, and laxatives.

Living inside a body that seems to be turning against you is difficult in more than one way. It is possible that the stress caused by the condition can actually make it worse. In some cases, counseling and antidepressants may be appropriate. And some conditions can be improved by surgery, to improve the way the gut works or to remove blockages from the intestines.

For many suffering from digestive disorders, a low-FODMAP diet is able to alleviate these symptoms without any medications or their aggravating side effects. More and more, doctors are recommending the low-FODMAP diet for their patients. They may even suggest consultation with a dietitian or nutritionist, because the diet represents a significant change in terms of the foods you cook and eat. And motivation is built into this diet, because many people report feeling better very quickly.

A FODMAP diet consists of an initial phase, sometimes called the acute phase or elimination phase. The purpose of this stage, which usually lasts two weeks, is to give your digestive system a chance to reset. During this stage, the aim is to avoid foods that are high in FODMAPs. Fruits, for example, are limited on the diet, and serving sizes and how often you eat them are controlled. There are suggested serving sizes for fresh and dried fruits, as well as some moderate FODMAP vegetables like sweet potatoes. It can be challenging to stick to a menu that is perhaps less varied than you are used to, but this stage is important for getting your body back to feeling good and being healthy.

Once you have completed the acute phase, you reintroduce foods in a series of controlled "challenges." In this phase, you gradually expand your food options with selections and quantities that are comfortable for you. Some people find that they can tolerate garlic, for instance, as long as it isn't consumed more than once a day; for others, garlic may remain a problem.

The challenges phase of the diet is set up in a systematic fashion, over two or three days, with each challenge separated from another by about four days. Through this process, you will find a new world of foods which you once thought were a problems are now a safe and delicious part of your diet. It is not uncommon for someone who suspects he or she is are lactose-intolerant to find out that milk is not a trigger food.

On the first day of the challenge, you add a small amount, about half a serving, of a high-FODMAP food from the group you are investigating. If you have a reaction from a small amount, you stop the challenge and return to the acute phase diet for three or four days before starting the next challenge. But if you do not react to a small serving, the next day, you have a larger serving and observe your reaction. If you can tolerate the food, you can reintroduce it to your diet safely, as long as you don't overdo it in terms of the frequency or size of the servings. Then you move on to the next challenge, and so on, until you have identified all the FODMAP foods that are appropriate for you and those that are not.

Food Sources with High FODMAPs

Fructans	Wheat, rye, onions, garlic, asparagus, artichokes, snow peas
Galactans (GOS)	Legumes (chickpeas, lentils, navy beans, pinto beans, black beans, soybeans, black-eyed peas, etc.)
Lactose	Milk, yogurt, soft or fresh cheeses (ricotta, cottage cheese)
Fructose	Honey, apples, pears, watermelon, mango, cherries
Polyols	Apples, pears, stone fruits, mushrooms, cauliflower, sugar-free mints and gums

As you continue the process, you may find that certain groups of foods, such as those containing high amounts of fructans or galactans, or polyols, are particular problems for you. Some foods contain more than one type of sachharide or polyol. You should introduce any new food to your diet cautiously, as you would in a challenge, to determine whether and how much you can tolerate.

A low-FODMAP diet can be healthy and delicious. The point of an elimination diet is to eventually reintroduce as many foods as you can tolerate. A long-term diet that excludes a wide range of foods is usually impossible to follow. And there is a danger that you might end up deficient in some important nutrients. The aim of the low-FODMAPS diet is to recondition your digestive system and to identify foods you can tolerate and enjoy over a lifetime.

CHAPTER TWO

FODMAPs, Food, and You

As you've noticed from the lists in the previous chapter, a food can be healthful, natural, free-range, or organic and still be considered a high-FODMAP food, right along with a number of foods of dubious nutritional value. FODMAPs are simply part of the structure of fruits, grains, vegetables, milk, and honey.

Why the Low-FODMAP Diet Works

The low-FODMAP diet works by identifying the foods that are problems for you to absorb and helping you avoid them in irritating quantities. When your body is constantly assaulted by high-FODMAP foods, your entire digestive system has to work very hard, but it isn't working very effectively because it is irritated and inflamed. Once the irritants are removed, as they are on the initial stage of a FODMAP diet, your system can calm down. When that happens, you can start to see the distinction between how a specific food makes you feel, rather than feeling generally horrible no matter what you eat. You learn to determine, for example, if it was the glass of milk that gave you problems or the whole grain cereal you poured it over for breakfast.

The first phase of the diet is challenging because it requires monitoring and planning, and because you have a rather short list of suitable foods to eat across a wide range of categories. But by taking advantage of the planning and observing aspects of the diet, you lay the groundwork for moving back into an eating pattern that is rich and varied. For some people, the effects are so positive that they actually limit themselves from more foods than they need to, because they are all too aware of what can happen if they eat something that does not agree with them.

Is the Low-FODMAP Diet Right for You?

Everyone's situation is different, and the low-FODMAP diet can adapt to a wide range of possibilities. Here are some common questions you may have about the plan.

I prefer to follow a vegetarian diet. Is this diet safe for me?

Finding a variety of foods during the first few weeks of the diet is challenging for everyone, but vegetarians may be especially challenged in finding adequate protein. If you are a lacto-ovo vegetarian and can include eggs and cheese, getting enough protein is not a problem. There are many plant-based protein foods that you can choose from, including nuts and peanuts. Seitan, made from vital wheat gluten, is another option.

Can I lose weight on the low-FODMAP diet?

Some foods on the low-FODMAP diet are consumed in small quantities. This kind of portion awareness is a good start for weight loss. You can adjust serving sizes to keep calories under control, as long as you don't restrict yourself too severely. Be sure you are eating enough to maintain your overall health and energy levels. Many people report that they do lose weight on the low-FODMAP plan without planning to do so. Whether that is because they are simply paying more attention to what they eat or because the inflammation and water-retention in the gut diminishes is hard to establish.

Is the low-FODMAP diet the same thing as a gluten-free diet?

No. Someone with gluten intolerance, like celiac disease, must strictly avoid wheat, rye, and barley. These grains do contain gluten. However, gluten itself is not a FODMAP food. Looking for gluten-free versions of pastas, cereals, and crackers is a good way to avoid some FODMAPs, but that is because "gluten-free" usually signals "wheat-free" as well. As long as you do not have a specific intolerance to gluten, it is the wheat you need to avoid, not the gluten.

I have lactose intolerance, but there seems to be dairy and cheese on many low-FODMAP plans. Why are some quantities of dairy included?

Milk sugar, or lactose, is a significant part of milk and is a FODMAP item. However, when milk is processed into butter, cheese, and cream, the watery portion of the milk, which contains the lactose, is reduced to a level that usually is not a problem. In the case of cultured milks and creams, like yogurt, kefir, and buttermilk, it is best to look for lactose-free alternatives, although some studies show that traditionally cultured yogurt and kefir, made with a specific bacterial culture, actually predigest the lactose, making it safe for some people.

I have celiac disease. Is there anything special I should know about the low-FODMAP diet?

Celiac disease is a serious condition that requires medical care and monitoring. The disease actually attacks the lining of the intestine and damages it. Someone with celiac disease must avoid all gluten to prevent further damage. If you have celiac disease, you must be vigilant about avoiding gluten, so some foods on the low-FODMAP plan may not be suitable for you.

When I read about FODMAPs, I get conflicting information about foods that are and are not considered low-FODMAP items. Why is that happening?

More and more foods are being evaluated for the quantity and type of FODMAPs they contain. As information becomes available, it is released. Sometimes it supports previous information, sometimes it contradicts it. In addition, people with IBS and similar conditions, especially, have to take a very personal approach to controlling what and how they eat. Books and websites based on personal experience with FODMAPs have some valuable information, but always regard online anecdotal statements with caution. A third consideration is that foods are not as uniform as you might imagine. One beet is quite different from another, so likewise, some people find a certain food tolerable on a low-FODMAP diet while others do not. Response can depend on factors like the variety that was grown, the soil it grew in, how old the vegetable was when you ate it, and how much of it you consumed.

I have food allergies and sensitivities that already limit the foods I can safely eat. Will there be anything left to eat if I start a low-FODMAP diet?

The low-FODMAP diet is varied enough to adapt to such special concerns as milk or soy allergies, although the very early stages of the diet may seem a bit restrictive. Concentrate on foods you know you can eat without a problem and focus on finding simple, safe ways to add more flavor and color to dishes through herbs and spices.

Could there be FODMAPs in my medicines?

It is possible that your medications, even your vitamins and dietary supplements, contain FODMAPs, but if so, they are generally in such low quantities that they do not have any effect. However, if you are taking a number of different medications and you do have an allergy or intolerance, you should talk to your doctor or pharmacist to find out more about how your medicines are made and whether there are any safer alternatives.

CHAPTER THREE

Eating Without FODMAPs

If your doctor has suggested a low-FODMAP diet for you, you will discover that the diet takes a fresh and careful look at all of the foods you eat. Your dietary needs are not the same as someone else's. Your doctor may suggest that you work with a dietitian or nutritionist to help map out your plan, especially if you have other conditions that may further limit your food options, such as allergies or celiac disease.

During the first phase of a low-FODMAP diet, your food options will change dramatically. Some foods have a lot of substances like fructans, galactans, polyols, or lactose—high FODMAPs, in other words—while others have little or none of an offending substance—low FODMAPs. Many foods you may consider not only delicious but healthful are high-FODMAP foods. An apple a day may keep the doctor away if you have a healthy digestive system, but if you have a digestive disorder like IBS, it might send you into a serious gastrointestinal tailspin. Apples, onions, and garlic, among other foods, are considered healthful, but because of their fructans, for the time being they are foods you should avoid.

You should try eating small meals, spaced fairly regularly throughout the day. Eating large amounts of anything all at once can be disruptive while your system is still under siege. This tactic may take some advance planning, so you will find the menu plan in Chapter 4 a helpful guide.

A gluten-free diet is not the same thing as a low FODMAP diet, but when it comes to certain foods, seeing a "gluten-free" statement on a package in the grocery store can be of assistance. You'll still need to read the nutrition label, since there can be high FODMAPs in gluten-free foods, but you can often find appropriate alternatives for flours, grains, cereals, breads, and baked goods by focusing on those gluten-free foods when you shop.

Foods to Avoid, Foods to Enjoy

Researchers are learning more about FODMAPs, and foods are shifting from the excluded group to the included group. This can lead to confusion. Some FODMAP dietary guides include beets and broccoli, for example, while others exclude coconut and avocado. In the following lists, you will find foods that are currently considered foods to enjoy, foods to enjoy in moderation, and foods to avoid. Here are a few general guidelines to keep in mind:

- Limit alcohol intake and opt for clear spirits with sparkling water.

- Drink plenty of water.

- Eat in moderation.

- Chew your food well.

- Limit processed foods to cut down on hidden FODMAPs and irritants.

- Remember that fresh fruits, vegetables, meats, and fish are best.

Fruits

Use the following guidelines for fruits:

- Limit intake of suitable fruits to 1 serving per meal e.g., one banana or orange).

- Drink one-third to one-half a glass of suitable juice.

- An appropriate portion for berries or grapes is a small handful.

- An appropriate portion for suitable dried fruits is about 2 tablespoons (about 10 raisins).

- Choose unsweetened dried fruits (because many are coated in sugar).

Suitable Fruits

Bananas

Blueberries

Boysenberries

Cantaloupe

Cranberries

Grapefruit

Kiwis

Lemons

Limes

Mandarins

Oranges

Passion fruit

Pineapple

Rhubarb

Tangelos

Suitable Dried Fruits

Banana chips

Cranberries

Currants

Pineapple

Sultanas

Raisins

Fruits to Limit

Avocado

Grapes

Honeydew melon

Raspberries

Strawberries

Fruits to Avoid

Apple

Apricot

Blackberries

Cherries

Lychee

Mangoes

Nectarines

Peaches

Pears

Persimmons

Plums

Prunes

Watermelon

Vegetables

In the early stages of your low-FODMAP diet, stick to the suitable vegetables listed below. As you progress through the diet, you can begin to reintroduce others to your diet if you tolerate them easily. You'll find a few vegetables that are somewhat controversial, like avocados, in the recipes in this book. You should skip them entirely if they cause you trouble, but for most people, they are tolerated if you stay at or below the suggested serving size.

Suitable Vegetables

Alfalfa sprouts

Baby corn

Bamboo shoots

Bean shoots

Bok choy

Carrots

Celery

Chilis (hot)

Chinese cabbage (choy sum)

Corn

Cucumber

Eggplant

Endive

Ginger

Green beans

Green onions (green part only)

Lettuce

Olives

Parsnip

Peppers

Potatoes

Pumpkin

Rutabaga

Spinach

Squash

Taro

Tomato

Turnip

Yam

Zucchini

Vegetables to Limit

Beet

Broccoli

Vegetables to Avoid

Artichokes (globe and Jerusalem)

Asparagus

Broccoli

Brussels sprouts

Cabbage

Cauliflower

Chicory

Dandelion greens

Fennel

Garlic

Green onions (white part)

Leek

Mushrooms

Okra

Onions

Peas

Radicchio

Shallots

Snow peas

Sugar snap peas

Sweet potatoes

Dairy and Dairy Alternatives, and Cooking Fats

This food category includes milks, cheeses, cultured dairy products like yogurt and kefir, as well as cooking fats like butter and oil.

Suitable Dairy/Fats

Almond milk

Butter

Camembert and Brie cheese

Coconut milk

Custards and puddings made with lactose-free milk

Edam cheese

Eggs

Hard cheeses (like Parmesan)

Dairy-free ice cream substitutes (gelato, sorbet)

Lactose-free ice creams or desserts

Lactose-free milk

Lactose-free yogurt

Limburger cheese

Mozzarella

Parmesan

Provolone cheese

Rice milk

Romano cheese

Swiss cheese

Vegetable oils

Dairy/fats to limit or avoid

Buttermilk

Cream (light cream, half-and-half, whipping cream)

Cream cheese

Creamed soups

Evaporated milk

Fresh cheeses (e.g. ricotta, cottage cheese)

Ice cream

Milk, regular and low-fat milk (cow, goat, sheep)

Milk powder

Milk products (creamer, instant cocoa, etc.)

Processed cheese, cheese spreads

Puddings, custards

Regular and low-fat yogurt

Soft cheeses

Sour cream

Soy milk

Sweetened condensed milk

Yogurt, sweetened/flavored

What to Stock in Your Pantry

A low-FODMAP diet doesn't have to be bland or boring. There are plenty of ways to add flavor and excitement to your meals, whether you love Mexican, French, Italian, or Asian foods. Be sure to read all labels on any canned, bottled, or packaged foods to identify foods that you are trying to avoid and look for alternatives that are safe for you to eat during the acute phase of the diet. Here are some spices, herbs, and other ingredients that you can use to add flavor to your food and also a few important go-to items to stock in your pantry:

Basic Items

Anchovies

Canned tomatoes (whole and peeled, crushed, or diced; avoid tomato paste or products with tomato paste)

Canned tuna, salmon, or crab

Capers

Coconut milk

Fish sauce

Mustard

Oils including olive oil, nut oils, coconut oil, seed oils

Olives

Spices, whole and ground

Spice blends (check the label to look for any FODMAP ingredients)

Sun-dried tomatoes

Tamarind paste

Vinegar

Herbs

Fresh and dried herbs are a perfect way to add flavor without FODMAPs. The recipes in this book rely on the following:

basil

chives

mint

oregano

parsley

tarragon

Suitable Nuts and Seeds

Nuts and seeds are used widely in FODMAP cooking, as long as portion sizes are monitored. The only nuts you need to avoid are cashews and pistachios (although some plans permit these nuts).

Chia seed

Flaxseed

Almonds

Brazil nuts

Hazelnuts

Macadamia nuts

Peanuts

Pecans

Pine nuts

Pumpkin seeds

Sunflower seeds

Walnuts

Nut butters and seed butters (but avoid cashew and pistachio)

Sweeteners

You might be surprised to find that some FODMAP recipes call for regular white or brown sugar, but they can be appropriate as long as they are kept to a minimal level. Here are some other alternatives to try as a sweetener and in baked goods.

Suitable SAweeteners (in Limited and Controlled Amounts)

Golden syrup

Molasses

Maple syrup

White, brown, and raw

Suitable non-nutritive sweeteners such as stevia

Sweeteners to Avoid

Artificial sweeteners (see exceptions above)

Corn syrups

Corn syrup solids

Chicory root extract

High-fructose corn syrup

Honey

Inulin

Sugar-free or low-carb sweets, mints, gums, and dairy desserts

Soy Products

One area of concern is soy and soy products. Most experts on the low-FODMAP diet conclude that soy sauce and tofu are acceptable. Your own level of tolerance may be different, however, so use these foods with caution and eat only the recommended amounts. Sometimes, a few mouthfuls can make the difference between feeling fine and feeling awful.

Baking

Baking is probably one of the trickiest areas for someone following a low-FODMAP diet. It is hard to forego breads and pastries for weeks at a time. To make appropriate dishes while you are on the acute phase, you may want to stock up on a few specialty flours and thickeners. Most of the items in the following list are available in larger grocery stores as well as natural food stores. You can also find many of them online. If you are looking for more information about baking for a low-FODMAP diet, see the Resources, page 139. Here are a few of the items used in the recipes in this book:

Alternative Grains, Flours, and Thickeners

Amaranth

Arrowroot powder

Buckwheat

Coconut flour

Cornmeal

Gluten-free breads

Gluten-free cereals

Grits

Millet

Oats

Polenta

Potato flour

Quinoa

Rice flour

Sago

Sorghum

Tapioca

Teff flour

Xanthan gum

Wheat and Rye Products to Avoid

Barley (pearl and whole-grain)

Bread

Bread crumbs

Breakfast cereals

Bulgur wheat

Cakes and pastries

Cookies

Couscous

Crackers

Pasta and noodles

Rye (unless it is wheat-free; however most rye breads have significant amounts of wheat flour)

Semolina (contains wheat)

Cooking Methods and Equipment

Foods can be cooked by almost any technique you like, but it is a good idea to limit or avoid fried foods. They can be difficult for anyone to digest and have the effect of either slowing foods down or speeding them up on their way through your gut.

Since many people on the low-FODMAP diet miss the flavor of garlic and onions, garlic- and onion-infused creams and oils make a good alternative. Add the garlic or onion to the oil or cream, heat them together, and then take them from the heat to cool. While the oil or cream cools, the flavors are steeped into them so you get the flavor without the FODMAPs.

Basic Cooking Equipment

Blender (electric)

Colander

Cutting board

Food mill

Food processor

Grater or microplane

Immersion blender

Mandoline or Japanese slicer

Measuring cups, for liquids and for dry items

Measuring spoons

Mixing bowls

Rolling pin

Rubber scrapers

Salad spinner

Sharp knives

Sieve

Skillets, sauté pans, crêpe or omelet pan, saucepans, heavy sauce pot, soup or stock pot, roasting pans, roasting rack, cooling racks, loaf pans, casserole baking dishes, muffins tins, and cake pans

Spatulas

Spice grinder

Stand or hand electric mixer

Wooden spoons, for stirring

Dining Out on the Low-FODMAP Diet

To get the most out of the first stage of a FODMAP diet, you may find it easier to eat at home. But no matter what stage of the diet you are on, you should know the basic guidelines for eating out at restaurants.

- Choose a friendly cuisine. Asian cuisines (e.g., Chinese, Thai, Japanese, Korean, Indian, and Vietnamese) are usually rice-based, while Mediterranean cuisines are usually wheat-based.

- Avoid soups and stews that are made in large batches. These dishes almost always include onions and garlic that have been simmered in the dish.

- Ask for sauces and dressings on the side. You can control how much you use or skip it altogether.

- Order bottled water, plain or flavored seltzer, or tea instead of juices and sodas.

- Order grilled or broiled meats, fish, and poultry, served with the sauce on the side.

- Look for side dishes like baked potatoes or rice that are low-FODMAP items.

- Remember that the effects of FODMAPs are cumulative; you can "save up" a serving of a food like butter or cream to have when you are dining out.

- Hot cereals like oatmeal or simple egg dishes are good bets at breakfast, and are available even at fast-food outlets.

- Ask the waiter which dishes contain garlic, onions, or other foods that are problems for you and find out if they can be left out or if they are cooked into the dish.

- Salads are one of the easiest dishes to modify to remove FODMAPs.

- Sushi and sashimi are usually good choices for a low-FODMAP diet.

CHAPTER 4

14-Day Menu Plan

Week 1

Monday

Breakfast: Strawberry-Banana Smoothie (page 39) and a slice of
Pumpkin Bread (page 53)

Snack: Deviled Eggs (page 65)

Lunch: Escarole Soup (page 71)

Dinner: Pork and Eggplant Stir-Fry (page 108)
Steamed rice

Tuesday

Breakfast: Carrot Muffins (page 48)

Snack: 1 cup lactose-free or nut milk and 1 small piece of fruit

Lunch: Chef Salad (page 77)

Dinner: Crispy Tarragon Chicken (page 101)
Scalloped Potatoes (page 98)
Steamed green beans

Wednesday

Breakfast: Orange Cranberry Walnut Scones (page 46)

Snack: Granola (page 52) with lactose-free yogurt

Lunch: Panini (page 84)

Dinner: Cedar-Planked Salmon (page 118)

Green Rice (page 97)

Green salad with suitable vegetables

Thursday

Breakfast: Granola (page 52)

Snack: Stuffed Endive (page 62)

Lunch: Cobb Salad (page 76)

Dinner: Pan-Seared Flatiron Steak with Tapenade (page 109)

Polenta (page 96)

Sautéed Swiss Chard (page 94)

Friday

Breakfast: Dutch Baby (page 43) with Hash Browns (page 56)

Snack: Spiced Nuts (page 67)

Lunch: Turkey and Brie Sandwiches (page 85)

Dinner: Oat-Crusted Cod (page 116)

Green Rice (page 97)

Steamed green beans

Saturday

Breakfast: Oat and Almond Waffles (page 42)

Snack: Pickled carrots (page 66)

Lunch: Margherita "Pizzas" (page 64)

Dinner: Baked Spaghetti and Meatballs (page 115)

Green salad with suitable vegetables

Sunday

Breakfast: Poached Eggs (page 49) on Turkey Hash (page 55)

Snack: Sun-Dried Tomato "Hummus" (page 59) with Vegetable Chips (page 68)

Lunch: Reuben Sandwiches (page 86)

Dinner: Chicken Curry (page 102)

Green Rice (page 97)

Sautéed Swiss Chard (page 94)

Week 2

Monday

Breakfast: Pineapple Parfait (page 40)

Snack: Spiced Nuts (page 67)

Lunch: Caesar Salad (page 79)

Dinner: Meatloaf (page 113)

Scalloped Potatoes (page 98)

Steamed or boiled corn

Tuesday

Breakfast: Poached Eggs (page 49) and Hash Browns (page 56)

Snack: 1 cup lactose-free or nut milk and 1 small piece of fruit

Lunch: Tuna Melts (page 83)

Dinner: Chicken Saltimbocca (page 103)

Polenta (page 96)

Sautéed Swiss Chard (page 94)

Wednesday

Breakfast: Scrambled Eggs with Ham (page 50)

Snack: Stuffed Endive (page 62)

Lunch: Tortilla Soup (page 74)

Dinner: Shrimp Diavolo (page 120)

Green salad with suitable vegetables

Thursday

Breakfast: Grits with a breakfast steak (4 ounces)

Snack: Granola with lactose-free yogurt (page 52)

Lunch: Niçoise Salad (page 80)

Dinner: Vegetable Biryani (page 121)

Friday

Breakfast: Frittata with Spinach and Potato (page 51)

Snack: Sun-Dried Tomato "Hummus" (page 59) with Vegetable Chips (page 68)

Lunch: Spinach Salad (page 78)

Dinner: Chili con Carne (page 114)

Steamed rice

Saturday

Breakfast: Buckwheat Crêpes (page 41) filled with Scrambled Eggs with Ham (page 50)

Snack: Pickled Carrots (page 66)

Lunch: Minestrone (page 73)

Dinner: Lemon Parsley Stuffed Trout (page 117)

Green Rice (page 97)

Sunday

Breakfast: Almond French Toast (page 44)

1 cup lactose-free or nut milk and 1 small piece of fruit

Snack: Spiced Nuts (page 67)

Lunch: Tostadas (page 61)

Dinner: Navarin-Style Leg of Lamb (page 106)

PART TWO
Recipes

Breakfast

Strawberry-Banana Smoothie

Pineapple Parfait

Buckwheat Crêpes

Oat and Almond Waffles

Dutch Baby

Almond French Toast

Gluten-Free French Toast

Orange Cranberry Walnut Scones

Carrot Muffins

Poached Eggs

Scrambled Eggs with Ham

Frittata with Spinach and Potato

Granola

Pumpkin Bread

Grits

Turkey Hash

Hash Browns

Note: Recipes in boldface are suitable for the first stage of the FODMAP diet. Recipes in regular type contain an ingredient that is a moderate-FODMAP food; avoid eating these dishes within 3 hours of eating any other moderate FODMAP food, and limit portions.

Breakfast

If you like your breakfast short and simple, there are plenty of low-FODMAP options. Be sure to check the nutrition label if you're buying store-bought foods. Here are a few easy-to-stock-in-your-pantry breakfast cereals, both hot and cold:

- cornflakes
- muesli
- oatmeal
- buckwheat groats

Instead of toast or bagels, substitute corn tortillas. Replace regular or low-fat milk and yogurt with lactose-free versions, or nondairy milk and yogurt made from nuts and seeds (but not soy milk).

You can have fruits for breakfast too, as long as you have just one small piece (or half, if the fruit is very large) or no more than ¼ cup fresh berries:

- citrus (orange, tangerine, grapefruit)
- banana
- berries
- cantaloupe and honey-dew melon

Strawberry-Banana Smoothie

MAKES 2 SERVINGS

Moderate FODMAP

This smoothie is a quick and easy way to start your day. Add ground chia or flaxseed for a boost of protein.

1 cup crushed ice
½ cup almond milk
1 banana, sliced
6 strawberries, hulled and sliced

Combine all the ingredients in a blender and process until very smooth and frothy. Serve immediately.

Pineapple Parfait

Moderate FODMAP

If your yogurt is thin, you can drain it for a few hours in a coffee filter–lined strainer or colander. Draining yogurt makes it thicker and reduces the amount of lactose it contains.

1 cup Granola (page 52)
2 cups coconut yogurt
1 cup pineapple chunks

Layer the granola, yogurt, and pineapple in four parfait glasses or dishes. Serve immediately.

Buckwheat Crêpes

MAKES 8 CRÊPES; 4 SERVINGS

First Stage FODMAP

These crêpes are perfect all on their own or with a touch of butter and a squeeze of lemon or lime. You can also fill them with any of your favorites, including scrambled eggs or turkey hash.

4 large eggs
1 cup unsweetened almond milk
Pinch of sea salt
1 cup buckwheat flour
2 tablespoons coconut oil

1. Combine the eggs, almond milk, and salt. Add the buckwheat flour. Stir until smooth.

2. Heat a crêpe pan or a small sauté pan over medium high heat. Add enough coconut oil to coat the pan lightly.

3. Drop about $\frac{1}{3}$ cup batter into the pan. Swirl and tilt the pan to coat it evenly with the batter.

4. Reduce the heat to medium, and cook until the underside of the crêpe is golden, about 2 minutes. Flip the crêpe over with a spatula, and cook the second side for about 1 minute.

5. Transfer each crêpe to a platter and keep warm while cooking the remaining crêpes. Serve at once.

6. The crêpes can be made in advance. Separate the crêpes with parchment paper before wrapping and storing them. Store in the refrigerator for up to 3 days or in the freezer for up to 2 months.

Oat and Almond Waffles

MAKES 8 WAFFLES; 4 SERVINGS

Moderate FODMAP

Every waffle iron is a bit different. Be sure to allow plenty of time for the iron to preheat, and be generous with cooking spray or coconut oil, since this batter can stick a little more than wheat-based batters.

Cooking spray or coconut oil for waffle iron
1½ cups almond or coconut milk
1 large egg
¼ cup olive oil
1 cup rolled oats (gluten-free)
½ cup rice flour
½ cup chopped almonds
1 tablespoon baking powder
½ teaspoon sea salt

1. Preheat the waffle iron to medium-high heat. Spray the waffle iron with cooking spray or brush liberally with coconut oil.

2. Whisk together the almond milk, egg, and olive oil in a small bowl until smooth.

3. In a medium bowl, combine the oats, rice flour, almonds, baking powder, and salt. Add the egg mixture to the flour mixture, and stir until smooth.

4. For each waffle, drop about ⅓ cup batter onto the iron. Close the waffle iron and cook until golden and crisp on the outside and cooked through, 4 to 5 minutes. Repeat until all of the waffles are cooked.

5. Serve immediately.

Dutch Baby

Moderate FODMAP

Dutch babies are big, puffy, and airy. The coconut flour in this recipe holds up well, but the pancakes begin to deflate as soon as they come from the oven, so enjoy these on the weekend when you can call everyone to the table at the same time. Blueberries make a great low-FODMAP topping.

5 tablespoons unsalted butter or coconut oil
6 large eggs
1 cup almond milk or coconut milk
¼ teaspoon pure vanilla extract
1 cup almond flour or coconut flour
¼ teaspoon ground cinnamon
Lemon wedges for serving

1. Preheat the oven to 425°F.

2. Put the butter in a cast iron skillet and put the skillet in the oven while it heats. (It should be very hot when the pancake batter is added.)

3. Combine the eggs, almond milk, and vanilla in a medium bowl and whisk until smooth.

4. Blend the flour and cinnamon into the egg mixture and stir until smooth. Pour the batter carefully into the hot skillet.

5. Bake the pancake until the edges are puffed and light brown on the edges, about 25 minutes.

6. Cut the pancake into wedges and serve at once, accompanied with lemon wedges.

Breakfast

Almond French Toast

Moderate FODMAP

Some gluten-free breads are on the small side, so use more bread slices per person to make sure there's enough. If you remember the night before, set the bread out on a plate so it can harden slightly. It will soak up more of the custard for a great pudding consistency on the inside and a crisp golden exterior.

Custard
1 cup almond milk
4 large eggs, lightly beaten
²/₃ cup maple syrup
1 teaspoon pure vanilla extract
¼ teaspoon kosher salt

8 slices wheat-free gluten-free bread (stale is best)
¼ cup clarified butter
Confectioners' sugar, for garnish (optional)

44

The FODMAP Solution

1. To make the custard: In a wide, shallow bowl, combine the almond milk, eggs, maple syrup, vanilla, and salt. Whisk until smooth.

2. Dip the bread slices in the custard and transfer them to a baking sheet to rest while you heat the skillet.

3. Heat the butter in a large skillet over medium-high heat until it is hot but not smoking. Add the French toast slices to the pan in batches; they should not overlap. Cook until the underside is golden and slightly crisp, about 4 minutes. Turn once and finish on the second side until cooked through and golden, another 2 to 3 minutes. Adjust the heat under the skillet if necessary so the French toast cooks evenly without burning.

4. Serve at once, dusted with confectioner's sugar (if using).

Gluten-Free French Toast

MAKES 8 PIECES; 4 SERVINGS

Moderate FODMAP

Gluten-free breads respond well to being made into French toast. Put the bread slices on a cooling rack and let them dry out during the night before for the best texture.

Custard
2 cups lactose-free cow's milk or almond milk
4 large eggs
2 tablespoons maple syrup
2 teaspoons pure vanilla extract
½ teaspoon ground cinnamon

2 tablespoons butter or coconut oil
8 slices wheat-free, gluten-free bread

1. To make the custard: In a wide, shallow bowl, combine the milk, eggs, maple syrup, vanilla, and cinnamon with a whisk or fork until evenly blended.

2. Heat a large sauté pan or griddle over medium-high heat. Add enough of the butter or oil to coat the skillet liberally.

3. Add the bread slices to the custard. Turn to coat evenly on both sides.

4. Cook the French toast on the first side until golden brown, about 3 minutes. Turn once and cook on the second side until golden brown and cooked through, another 3 minutes.

5. Serve immediately.

Orange Cranberry Walnut Scones

MAKES 8 SCONES

Moderate FODMAP

You can keep the unbaked scones in the freezer for up to 2 months, if you like, and then bake them as you need them. Add about 10 minutes to the baking time for frozen scones.

Cooking spray, (optional)
2 cups almond flour
6 tablespoons arrowroot powder
2 teaspoons baking powder
½ teaspoon sea salt
¼ cup unsalted butter or coconut oil
1 large egg, lightly beaten
2 tablespoons maple syrup
Zest of 1 orange
3 tablespoons unsweetened dried cranberries

1. Preheat the oven to 350°F. Coat a baking sheet with cooking spray or line it with parchment paper.

2. In a medium bowl, combine the almond flour, arrowroot, baking powder, and salt with a whisk or fork.

3. Cut in the unsalted butter with a pastry cutter or two table knives until a crumbly meal forms with pieces of fat about the size of sesame seeds. Add the egg, maple syrup, orange zest, and cranberries. Mix with a fork just until evenly blended and moistened.

4. Scrape the batter onto a sheet of parchment paper. Top with a second sheet of parchment paper and press into an even disk about ½ inch thick and 9 inches wide.

5. Peel off the top sheet of parchment paper. Cut the disk into 8 equal wedges. Arrange the wedges on the prepared baking sheet, leaving about 2 inches between them. Bake until golden brown and baked through, 20 to 25 minutes.

6. Transfer the scones to a cooling rack.

7. Serve warm or at room temperature.

8. The scones can be prepared in advance. Store in an airtight container at room temperature for up to 2 days.

Carrot Muffins

Moderate FODMAP

These muffins are a portable breakfast item. If you make them in advance and freeze them, you can add one to a bagged lunch to keep things cool. By the time you are ready for lunch, the muffin will be thawed.

Coconut oil
½ cup almond flour
¼ cup coconut flour
1 tablespoon ground cinnamon
1 teaspoon ground nutmeg
¼ teaspoon sea salt
1 large ripe banana
4 large eggs, lightly beaten
1 cup grated carrots
1 tablespoon maple syrup
2 teaspoons pure vanilla extract

1. Preheat the oven to 350°F. Coat 12 muffin cups in two standard muffin tins lightly with coconut oil.

2. In a small bowl, whisk together the almond flour, coconut flour, cinnamon, nutmeg, and salt to combine thoroughly.

3. In a medium bowl, mash the banana with a fork until it is a smooth purée. Add the eggs, carrots, maple syrup, and vanilla.

4. Add the flour mixture to the banana mixture and stir to make a smooth batter. Spoon the batter into the muffin tins, filling them about three-fourths full.

5. Bake until the muffins spring back when lightly pressed in the center, 25 to 30 minutes.

6. Cool the muffins in the muffin tins for a few minutes before turning them out onto a rack. Keep muffins at room temperature in an airtight container for up to 3 days.

Poached Eggs

First Stage FODMAP

Poached eggs are perfect to put on top of Turkey Hash (page 55) or Hash Browns (page 56), or add them to one of the soups in Chapter 7 for a substantial lunch or supper.

2 tablespoons lemon juice
8 large eggs

1. Bring a pot of water to a gentle simmer over medium heat. Add the lemon juice.

2. Crack one of the eggs into a shallow dish or cup. Carefully pour the egg out of the dish into the simmering water. Work in batches to avoid crowding the pan or use two pots of water. Cook until the whites are set and the yolks are of the desired doneness, 4 to 5 minutes.

3. Lift the eggs from the water with a slotted spoon. Blot on paper towels.

4. Serve immediately.

49

Breakfast

Scrambled Eggs with Ham

First Stage FODMAP

Substitute other low-FODMAP meats for the ham or prosciutto, if you prefer, or leave it out completely in favor of a little aged cheese or some minced green onions. To make a breakfast burrito, roll the scrambled eggs in a warmed corn tortilla and top with some onion-free salsa.

4 large eggs
2 tablespoons water
Salt and freshly ground black pepper
2 tablespoons butter, olive oil, or coconut oil
3 tablespoons minced ham or prosciutto

1. In a medium bowl, combine the eggs and water and whisk until evenly blended. Season with salt and pepper.

2. Heat a medium sauté pan over medium-high heat. Add enough butter to coat the pan liberally.

3. Add the ham. Cook until crisp and browned, about 2 minutes. Add the beaten eggs to the skillet.

4. Cook the eggs, stirring frequently, until set into soft curds and fully cooked, 3 to 4 minutes.

5. Serve immediately.

Frittata with Spinach and Potato

MAKES 4 SERVINGS

First Stage FODMAP

Frozen spinach is great to have on hand in the freezer. To prepare it for this dish, let it thaw and then squeeze it in a strainer to remove as much extra water as possible.

2 tablespoons olive oil
1 cup diced cooked potatoes
2 cups chopped frozen spinach
Kosher salt and freshly ground black pepper
Pinch of freshly grated nutmeg
8 large eggs, beaten

1. Preheat the oven to 350°F.

2. Heat the olive oil in a cast-iron skillet over medium-high heat. Add the potatoes and sauté, stirring as necessary, until golden brown, 3 to 4 minutes. Add the spinach and sauté, stirring as necessary, until the spinach is very hot. Season with salt, pepper, and nutmeg.

3. Pour in the eggs.

4. Transfer the skillet to the oven and bake until the eggs are fully cooked, 20 to 25 minutes.

5. Serve immediately.

Breakfast

Granola

First Stage FODMAP

Granola is a favorite go-to breakfast cereal or snack. You can customize this recipe to include your favorite nuts (excluding pistachios and cashews) and seeds. Be careful with the dried fruits, however. The list of suitable dried fruits can be found on page 19.

4 ½ cups old-fashioned rolled oats (gluten-free)
⅔ cup coconut oil
½ cup maple syrup
½ cup chopped pecans
½ cup pumpkin seeds
¼ cup sunflower seeds
¼ cup sliced almonds
2 tablespoons finely grated orange zest

1. Preheat the oven to 325°F.

2. In a large bowl, combine all of the ingredients. Toss them together until evenly blended.

3. Spread the granola in an even layer on a parchment paper–lined baking sheet. Bake, stirring as necessary to brown evenly, until crunchy and toasted, about 1 hour.

4. Let the granola cool to room temperature. The granola can be stored in an airtight container at room temperature for up to 3 weeks.

Pumpkin Bread

MAKES 1 LOAF; 12 SERVINGS

Moderate FODMAP

Slice this bread and toast it in the morning and spread it with almond butter for a delicious and protein-packed breakfast that is perfect for busy mornings.

Cooking spray
1½ cups almond flour
¾ cup potato starch
½ cup cornstarch
1¼ teaspoon xanthan gum
2 teaspoon ground cinnamon
1 teaspoon sea salt
1 teaspoon baking soda
1 teaspoon baking powder
1 teaspoon ground ginger
¼ teaspoon ground nutmeg
1 cup pumpkin purée
1 cup maple syrup
½ cup canola oil
3 large eggs, lightly beaten
1 tablespoon pure vanilla extract
½ cup chopped walnuts or pecans (optional)

1. Preheat the oven to 375°F. Coat a loaf pan with cooking spray.

2. In a large bowl, combine the almond flour, potato starch, cornstarch, xanthan gum, cinnamon, salt, baking soda, baking powder, ginger, and nutmeg and whisk together.

3. In a small bowl, combine the pumpkin purée, maple syrup, oil, eggs, and vanilla and whisk until evenly blended.

4. Add the pumpkin mixture to the flour mixture, and stir until evenly combined. Stir in the nuts (if using).

5. Scrape the batter into the prepared loaf pan. Bake for 15 minutes and then reduce the heat to 325°F. Bake until golden brown and a toothpick inserted near the center of the loaf comes out clean, with a few moist crumbs clinging, 45 to 50 minutes.

6. Cool the bread completely on a wire rack before slicing and serving.

Grits

First Stage FODMAP

A classic dish from the South, grits make a rich and satisfying cereal, or you can use them as a base for poached eggs, sausage, or ham.

4 cups water
¾ teaspoon sea salt
¾ cup yellow cornmeal
¾ cup grated aged Cheddar cheese (optional)

1. In a large saucepan, bring the water and ¾ teaspoon salt to a simmer over medium-high heat.

2. Add the cornmeal, a few tablespoons at a time, stirring constantly, until all has been added. Reduce the heat to low and simmer, stirring constantly, until thickened and creamy, 15 to 20 minutes.

3. Add the Cheddar cheese (if using). Season again with salt, if desired.

4. Serve immediately.

Turkey Hash

First Stage FODMAP

If you have fresh or dried cranberries on hand, add a few to this dish and it is Thanksgiving all over again.

2 tablespoons olive oil or canola oil
2 cups diced cooked potatoes
1 cup diced cooked parsnips
½ cup grated carrots
½ cup minced green onions
12 ounces diced cooked turkey
½ teaspoon fresh thyme leaves
Kosher salt and freshly ground black pepper

1. Heat the oil in a large cast-iron skillet over medium-high heat.

2. Add the potatoes, parsnips, carrots, and green onions. Sauté, stirring frequently, until the potatoes are coated with oil and beginning to turn golden, 4 to 5 minutes.

3. Add the turkey and thyme, and season with salt and pepper. Continue to cook without stirring until a crust develops on the bottom of the hash, 6 to 8 minutes. Turn the hash with a wide spatula, lifting large sections at a time to keep as much of the crust intact as possible.

4. Cook on the second side until a crust develops, an additional 5 to 6 minutes. Cut into wedges.

5. Serve immediately.

Hash Browns

First Stage FODMAP

Make this dish as one large cake to cut into wedges, as this recipe suggests, or shape them into smaller, individual patties.

2 tablespoons olive oil or clarified butter (or ghee), plus
      more as needed
3 cups shredded potatoes
3 tablespoons chopped fresh chives
1 teaspoon fresh thyme leaves (or ½ teaspoon dried)
Kosher salt and freshly ground black pepper

1. Heat the oil in a large cast-iron skillet over medium-high heat. Add half of the potatoes and press into an even layer. Sprinkle the chives and thyme evenly over the potatoes, and season with salt and pepper. Top with the remaining potatoes. Drizzle with a little additional oil.

2. Cook on the first side without stirring until a crust develops on the bottom, 6 to 8 minutes. Turn the potatoes with a wide spatula, lifting large sections at a time to keep as much of the crust intact as possible.

3. Cook on the second side until a crust develops, an additional 5 to 6 minutes. Cut into wedges.

4. Serve immediately.

Snacks

Note: Recipes in boldface are suitable for the first stage of the FODMAP diet. Recipes in regular type contain an ingredient that is a moderate FODMAP. Avoid eating these dishes within 3 hours of eating any other moderate FODMAP food, and limit portions.

Snacks

When you are on the low-FODMAP diet, it is a good idea to be ready for snack time. Planning ahead helps you avoid grabbing foods not on your plan. And it also gives you a chance to prepare for several small meals throughout the day rather than a few large ones, which will help you digest your food properly.

If you are looking for simple snack ideas, consider the following:

- aged cheese
- dried fruit
- glass of lactose-free or nut milk
- hard-cooked eggs
- jerky
- nuts

- piece of suitable fresh fruit (banana, small orange, or other)
- popcorn
- raw vegetables
- trail mix
- yogurt (lactose-free)

Sun-Dried Tomato "Hummus"

MAKES 2 CUPS; 4 TO 5 SERVINGS

First Stage FODMAP

Use this as a dip or a spread. It is delicious with vegetables as well as on grilled or sautéed meats, and it keeps well in the refrigerator.

1 cup oil-packed sun-dried tomatoes, with their oil
1 cup shredded zucchini
½ cup coarsely chopped fresh cilantro leaves
¼ cup tahini
2 tablespoons lemon juice, plus more as needed
2 tablespoons water, plus more as needed
2 tablespoons olive oil, plus additional for serving
1 teaspoon dark sesame oil
Kosher salt and freshly ground black pepper

1. Combine the sun-dried tomatoes and their oil, zucchini, cilantro, and tahini in a food processor. Purée until the mixture becomes a coarse paste, scraping down the bowl if necessary.

2. Add the lemon juice, water, olive oil, and sesame oil through the feed tube with the machine running. Purée the mixture until it becomes a smooth paste. Adjust the consistency with additional water, if necessary. Adjust the seasoning with additional lemon juice if necessary, and season with salt and pepper.

3. Serve immediately or store the hummus in a covered container in the refrigerator for up to 4 days.

Snacks

Garlic-Infused Oil

MAKES 1 CUP

First Stage FODMAP

Use this basic technique to make onion-infused oil with the white portion of green onions, shallots, or even leeks to flavor your foods and to use in cooking. Store the oil in the refrigerator; the oil has a limited shelf life, so make an amount you can use within a week. Dip gluten-free bread into the oil for a light snack.

1 cup olive oil
8 garlic cloves peeled and crushed
1 teaspoon red pepper flakes (optional)

1. Heat the oil in a heavy-gauge pot over medium heat. Add the garlic and red pepper flakes (if using). Cook until aromatic, 2 to 3 minutes.

2. Remove from the heat. Let cool to room temperature.

3. Strain the oil into a clean jar. Discard the garlic and red pepper flakes.

4. Store the oil in the refrigerator for up to 7 days.

Tostadas

First Stage FODMAP

Instead of turkey, you can use other ground meats, like beef, lamb, pork, sausage, or venison, if you prefer. This recipe is a great build-your-own snack. You can always put out other toppings if your friends and family aren't following the FODMAP diet, but they may not notice that anything is missing.

1 tablespoon olive oil
1 pound lean ground turkey
2 teaspoons chili powder (garlic-free)
1 teaspoon ground cumin
1 cup diced tomatoes (canned or fresh)
Salt and freshly ground black pepper
8 tostada shells (gluten-free)
1 cup grated aged sharp Cheddar cheese
2 green onions (green part only), minced

1. Preheat the oven to 325°F. Heat the oil in a large cast-iron skillet over high heat. Add the ground turkey. Sauté, stirring frequently, until the meat is evenly cooked and browned, 6 to 8 minutes. Add the chili powder and cumin, and stir to combine. Add the tomatoes. Cook, stirring occasionally, until thickened and flavorful, 10 to 12 minutes. Season with salt and pepper.

2. Place the tostada shells on two baking sheets. Divide the turkey mixture, cheese, and green onions evenly among the shells. Bake until the cheese is melted and bubbly, 8 to 10 minutes.

3. Serve immediately.

Stuffed Endive

MAKES 8 SPEARS; 4 SERVINGS

Moderate FODMAP

Look for red endive to make a really stunning hors d'oeuvre.

12 ounces Brie or Camembert cheese, rind removed
2 green onions (green part only), minced
8 leaves Belgian endive
½ cup minced fresh flat-leaf parsley or fresh chives
Freshly ground black pepper

1. Blend the Brie and green onions in a medium bowl with a wooden spoon or in a food processor until evenly combined.

2. Fill the endive leaves with the Brie-onion mixture. Sprinkle with parsley and season with pepper.

3. Serve immediately.

Flatbreads for Pizza

MAKES 4 FLATBREADS

Moderate FODMAP

*These flatbreads have many uses beyond pizza. You can simply enjoy
them as a bread to accompany a soup or stew. Or if you prefer, fill them
with your favorite sandwich items and griddle them to make toasted
sandwiches or panini.*

1½ cups oat flour, plus more for rolling
⅔ cups tapioca flour
¼ cups brown rice flour
½ teaspoon baking powder
½ teaspoon sea salt
½ cup almond milk
2 teaspoons lemon juice
2 teaspoons minced rosemary (optional)
½ teaspoon freshly ground black pepper (optional)
2 teaspoons clarified butter or ghee

1. In a large bowl, combine the oat flour, tapioca flour, brown rice flour,
baking powder, and salt.

2. In a small bowl, combine the almond milk and lemon juice, and let sit for
a few minutes to curdle.

3. To the flour mixture, add the curdled milk, rosemary (if using), and
pepper (if using) and stir to make a stiff dough.

4. Divide the dough into four equal pieces. Working with one piece of dough
at a time, roll out into disks on a well-floured work surface with a rolling pin,
about ½ inch thick and 7 or 8 inches in diameter. Coat the dough and rolling
pin with additional oat flour as needed to prevent sticking.

5. Heat the clarified butter in a large cast-iron skillet over medium-high
heat. Add one flatbread to the skillet. Cook on the first side until golden
brown, 6 to 7 minutes. Turn and cook on the second side until golden brown
and cooked through, 2 to 3 minutes. Repeat with the remaining flatbreads.

6. Serve immediately. The flatbreads can be prepared in advance. Store in an
airtight container in the refrigerator for up to 3 days or in the freezer for up
to 2 months.

Snacks

Margherita "Pizzas"

Moderate FODMAP

Let fresh mozzarella drain before you put it on the pizza—for two reasons: the pizza will be crisper and the mozzarella will have even less lactose.

4 Flatbreads for Pizza (page 63)
2 cups tomato sauce
4 ounces fresh mozzarella, sliced and drained
¼ cup coarsely chopped fresh basil
2 tablespoons grated Parmesan cheese
1 tablespoon olive oil or Garlic-Infused Oil (page 60)

1. Preheat the oven to 425°F.

2. Place the flatbreads on baking sheets. Top with the tomato sauce, mozzarella, basil, Parmesan, and olive oil.

3. Bake until the cheese is melted and golden, 10 to 12 minutes. Serve immediately.

Deviled Eggs

MAKES 12 HALVES; 4 SERVINGS

First Stage FODMAP

A favorite at picnics and gatherings, deviled eggs are also low-FODMAP items. Be sure your mayonnaise doesn't contain added sugar or syrup. The technique for hard-cooking eggs is very reliable, as long as you pay attention to when the water comes to a boil. They emerge from the shells fully cooked and tender, with no green rings around the yolk.

6 large eggs
¼ cup mayonnaise
1 tablespoon mustard
Pinch of cayenne pepper
Kosher salt and freshly ground black pepper
Paprika, for garnish
Minced fresh chives, for garnish

1. Put the eggs in a large saucepan. Add enough cold water to cover by 2 inches.

2. Bring to a boil over medium-high heat. Turn off the heat. Cover the pot. Let the eggs sit in the hot water for 15 minutes. Drain the water. When the eggs are cool enough to handle, peel them and cut in half. Separate the yolks from the whites: place the whites on a platter and the yolks in a medium bowl.

3. To the egg yolks, add the mayonnaise, mustard, and cayenne. Mash the egg yolk mixture with a fork until very smooth and light. Season with salt and pepper. Fill the egg whites evenly with the yolk mixture.

4. Sprinkle with paprika and chives for garnish. Serve immediately.

5. The eggs can be cooked in advance. Peel the eggs before storing. Store in a covered container in the refrigerator for up to 3 days.

Pickled Carrots

First Stage FODMAP

These spicy-sweet-sour carrots are addictive, just like potato chips. You can make a double batch and keep them on hand; they last for several days in the refrigerator, getting even more flavorful as they rest.

3 cups water, plus more as needed
1 cup red wine vinegar
2 teaspoons sea salt
¼ teaspoon red pepper flakes
1 pound baby carrots or carrots cut into sticks

1. Combine the water, vinegar, salt, and red pepper flakes in a large bowl or a glass jar. Stir until the salt dissolves. Add the carrots to the bowl. Add more water if necessary to completely submerge the carrots.

2. Marinate in the refrigerator at least 24 hours and up to 4 days before serving.

Spiced Nuts

Moderate FODMAP

Nuts are a great snack, but remember to keep them to a small portion size, about ¼ cup or a small handful. Keep these nuts on hand in an airtight container, or make a lot to take along to parties and events where you might find yourself tempted.

4 ounces almonds
4 ounces walnuts
4 ounces pecans
1 tablespoon olive oil
2 teaspoons chili powder
1 teaspoons ground cumin
Kosher salt and freshly ground black pepper

1. Preheat the oven to 350°F.

2. In a medium bowl, combine all of the ingredients and toss until evenly coated. Transfer the nuts to a rimmed baking sheet and spread them out in an even layer.

3. Bake, stirring occasionally to brown evenly, until toasted and golden, 10 to 12 minutes. Transfer the nuts to a container.

4. Store the spiced nuts in an airtight container at room temperature for up to 2 weeks.

Vegetable Chips

MAKES 1 POUND; 8 SERVINGS

First Stage FODMAP

Use a mandoline or Japanese slicer to make paper-thin slices that get crispy and golden as they bake. Add minced fresh herbs, ground spices, or a little Parmesan cheese along with the oil, if you like, for flavor variations.

2 pounds thinly sliced zucchini or Japanese eggplant
2 tablespoons olive oil or Garlic-Infused Oil (page 60)
Kosher salt

1. Preheat the oven to 425°F.

2. In a large bowl, combine the zucchini and olive oil and toss until evenly coated. Transfer to a rimmed baking sheet.

3. Bake, turning occasionally to crisp evenly, until toasted and crisp, 15 to 16 minutes. Season with salt while the chips are still very hot.

4. Serve immediately.

Soups, Salads, and Sandwiches

Escarole Soup

Tomato Bisque

Minestrone

Tortilla Soup

Corn and Potato Chowder

Cobb Salad

Chef Salad

Spinach Salad

Caesar Salad

Niçoise Salad

Mediterranean Salad

Sloppy Joes

Tuna Melts

Panini

Turkey and Brie Sandwiches

Reuben Sandwiches

Note: Recipes in boldface are suitable for the first stage of the FODMAP diet. Recipes in regular type contain an ingredient that is a moderate FODMAP. Avoid eating these dishes within 3 hours of eating any other moderate FODMAP food, and limit portions.

CHAPTER SEVEN

Soups, Salads, and Sandwiches

You can build lunches and dinners around the recipes in this chapter by serving any suitable vegetables along with a salad or soup. If you are adding a moderate FODMAP ingredient, remember to observe the portion size in the recipe, especially during the acute phase of the diet.

For quick and easy sandwiches and salads that you can put together from your pantry and fridge, be sure to have foods like these on hand:

- Thinly sliced deli meats (make sure they are gluten-free)

- Canned tuna or salmon (check the label to be sure it does not contain high fructose corn syrup)

- Gluten-free bread or tortillas

- Traditionally fermented pickles

- Hardboiled eggs

- Lactose-free or non-dairy yogurt (unsweetened)

- Leafy greens

- Fresh, seasonal vegetables from the suitable list (page 20)

- Broths and stocks (homemade, without onions or garlic)

Escarole Soup

Moderate FODMAP

To this soup, add shredded or cubed cooked meats or sliced, spicy sausage for a more substantial dish (check the label to be sure any cured meats are low-FODMAP items). For a kick, use Garlic-Infused Oil (page 60).

1 tablespoon olive oil
½ cup thinly sliced carrots
¾ cup diced potatoes
12 ounces escarole, chopped
6 cups chicken or vegetable broth
2 cups diced tomatoes with their juice
1 dried bay leaf
1 sprig fresh thyme
Kosher salt and freshly ground black pepper

1. Heat the olive oil in a soup pot over medium-high heat. Add the carrots and potatoes, and sauté until the vegetables are just starting to brown, 3 to 4 minutes. Add the escarole. Cook, stirring frequently, until the escarole is wilted and bright green, 4 to 5 minutes.

2. Add the broth, tomatoes, bay leaf, and thyme sprig. Season with salt and pepper, and stir to combine. Reduce the heat to medium-low, and simmer until the vegetables are tender and the soup is flavorful, 30 to 35 minutes. Remove and discard the bay leaf and thyme.

3. Serve in heated soup bowls.

Soups, Salads, and Sandwiches

Tomato Bisque

Moderate FODMAP

Instead of relying on flour and cream to make a thick tomato bisque, this recipe relies on rice. Rice is traditionally used in soups to add body and thickness. Be sure to let the rice cook until it is nearly falling apart.

1 tablespoon oil
½ cup minced green onions, green portion only
¾ cup carrots
½ cup long-grain rice
3 cups diced tomatoes
6 cups chicken or vegetable broth
6 fresh flat-leaf parsley sprigs
1 sprig fresh thyme
Kosher salt and freshly ground black pepper
Minced fresh parsley, chives, or thyme, for garnish

1. Heat the oil in a soup pot over medium-high heat. Add the green onions and carrots. Sauté, stirring occasionally, until the green onions are bright green and the carrots are tender, 3 to 4 minutes. Add the rice, tomatoes, broth, parsley sprigs, and thyme sprig. Season with salt and pepper, and stir to combine.

2. Reduce the heat to medium-low and simmer until the rice is very tender and the soup is flavorful, 25 to 30 minutes. Remove and discard the parsley and thyme sprigs.

3. Purée the soup with an immersion blender directly in the pot or let it cool for 10 minutes and then purée in a blender or food processor.

4. Just before serving, return the soup to a simmer and stir in the chopped herbs. Serve in warmed bowls.

Minestrone

MAKES 6 TO 8 SERVINGS

Moderate FODMAP

This fragrant, delicious soup takes a few liberties with the classic recipe: walnuts replace the beans, rice vermicelli replaces wheat pasta, and green onions (just the tops!) add the sharp flavors you expect. If you are using canned tomatoes, check the label to avoid added sugar.

1 tablespoon olive oil
½ cup minced green onions, green portion only
1 celery stalk, thinly sliced
1 teaspoon dried oregano
1 teaspoon dried basil
1½ cups tomatoes with their juice
6 cups chicken or vegetable broth
1 dried bay leaf
2 sprigs fresh oregano or basil
12 ounces chopped fresh kale
9 ounces rice vermicelli
¼ cup chopped walnuts
½ cup grated Parmesan cheese
Kosher salt and freshly ground black pepper

1. Heat the olive oil in a soup pot over medium-high heat. Add the green onions, celery, oregano, and basil. Sauté, stirring occasionally, until the vegetables are bright green and tender, 4 to 5 minutes.

2. Add the tomatoes, broth, bay leaf, and sprigs of oregano, and stir to combine. Reduce the heat to medium-low and simmer until the soup is flavorful, 12 to 14 minutes.

3. Add the kale, vermicelli, and walnuts. Simmer until the kale and vermicelli are fully cooked and tender, 12 to 14 minutes. Remove and discard the bay leaf and oregano sprigs.

4. Just before serving, return the soup to a simmer. Stir in the Parmesan and season with salt and pepper.

5. Serve in warmed bowls.

Tortilla Soup

Moderate FODMAP

If you want some heat in the broth without adding chilis directly to the soup, add some red pepper flakes along with the chili powder and cumin.

6 yellow corn tortillas, cut into strips
1 tablespoon olive oil
½ cup minced green onions, green portion only
2 teaspoons chili powder
1 teaspoon ground cumin
1 cup diced tomatoes with their juice
6 cups chicken or vegetable broth
6 fresh cilantro sprigs
Kosher salt and freshly ground black pepper
8 ounces shredded or diced cooked chicken
¼ cup chopped fresh cilantro
1 tablespoon lime juice
1 lime sliced into 6 wedges

1. Preheat the oven to 350°F.

2. Put the tortillas on a baking sheet. Bake until crisp and golden, 15 to 20 minutes. Cool to room temperature. Crumble half of the tortilla strips into pieces. Reserve the remaining tortilla strips for garnish.

3. Heat the olive oil in a soup pot over medium-high heat. Add the green onions, crumbled tortillas, chili powder, and cumin. Sauté, stirring occasionally, until the green onions are bright green, 2 to 3 minutes. Add the tomatoes, broth, and cilantro sprigs. Season with salt and pepper.

4. Reduce the heat to medium-low, and simmer until all of the ingredients are tender and the soup is flavorful, 25 to 30 minutes. Remove and discard the cilantro sprigs. Purée the soup with an immersion blender directly in the pot, or let it cool for 10 minutes and then purée in a blender or food processor.

5. Just before serving, return the soup to a simmer and stir in the chicken, chopped cilantro, and lime juice.

6. Serve in warmed bowls with tortilla strips and lime wedges.

Corn and Potato Chowder

Moderate FODMAP

Manhattan-style chowder, made with broth and tomatoes, is the inspiration for this soup. To make this a main course chowder, add chunks of fish fillets, scallops, clams, lobster, or shrimp.

1 tablespoon olive oil
2 cups diced peeled potatoes
2 celery stalks, thinly sliced
2 cups corn kernels, fresh or thawed frozen
6 cups chicken or vegetable broth
2 cups diced tomatoes with their juice
1 sprig fresh thyme
1 dried bay leaf
Kosher salt and freshly ground black pepper
¼ cup thinly sliced green onions, green portion only

1. Heat the olive oil in a soup pot over medium-high heat. Add the potatoes, celery, and corn.

2. Sauté, stirring occasionally, until the vegetables just start to brown, 8 to 10 minutes.

3. Add the broth, tomatoes, thyme sprig, and bay leaf, and season with salt and pepper. Stir to combine. Reduce the heat to medium-low, and simmer until the vegetables are tender and the soup is flavorful, 25 to 30 minutes. Remove and discard the thyme and bay leaf.

4. Just before serving, return the soup to a simmer and stir in the green onions. Serve in warmed bowls.

Cobb Salad

Moderate FODMAP

A classic Cobb salad includes plenty of FODMAP-friendly ingredients, with the possible exception of avocado. This recipe reins in the quantity of avocado to a manageable amount, so be sure you don't exceed the listed quantities (but do add the rest of the avocado to someone else's salad, or try it for a facial, if there's no one to eat it up).

¼ cup olive oil
2 tablespoons lemon juice
1 teaspoon Dijon mustard
Kosher salt and freshly ground black pepper

4 cups mixed salad greens
12 ounces cooked turkey, sliced
4 strips nitrate-free bacon, cooked and crumbled
8 thin slices avocado (optional)
4 ounces blue cheese, crumbled
2 tomatoes, cut into wedges
½ cup diced peeled cucumber

1. To make the dressing, in a small bowl, whisk together the olive oil, lemon juice, and mustard and season with salt and pepper. Set aside.

2. On individual plates or a platter, make a bed of the mixed salad greens. Arrange the turkey, bacon, avocado (if using), blue cheese, tomato wedges, and cucumber on the salad greens.

3. Serve at once, with the dressing to pour over.

Chef Salad

Moderate FODMAP

A good chef salad is the perfect way to make a satisfying lunch or light dinner without having to turn on the stove. Do research on the brands of deli meats you buy; some may include ingredients derived from such high-FODMAPs as milk or whey.

¼ cup olive oil
2 tablespoons lemon juice
1 teaspoon Dijon mustard
1 teaspoon minced fresh tarragon or ½ teaspoon dried tarragon
Kosher salt and freshly ground black pepper

6 cups mixed salad greens
4 ounces sliced turkey
4 ounces sliced ham
4 ounces sliced roast beef
4 ounces sliced Swiss cheese
2 tomatoes, cut into wedges
2 hard-cooked eggs, cut into wedges

1. To make the dressing, in a small bowl, combine the oil, lemon juice, mustard, and tarragon, and season with salt and pepper. Set aside.

2. On individual plates or a platter, make a bed of the salad greens. Arrange the turkey, ham, roast beef, Swiss cheese, tomato wedges, and eggs on the greens.

3. Serve at once, accompanied by the dressing.

Spinach Salad

Moderate FODMAP

Marinated or seasoned tofu is used here to replace the texture and flavor of more traditional but high-FODMAP mushrooms, which should be avoided during the elimination phase of your diet. Tofu does come from beans, but because of its processing, it has been included on the list of foods appropriate for this diet.

¼ cup olive oil
2 tablespoons orange juice
1 teaspoon orange zest
1 teaspoon minced fresh chives
Kosher salt and freshly ground black pepper
6 cups gently packed baby spinach
½ cup cubed marinated tofu
2 tomatoes, cut into wedges
2 hard-cooked eggs, cut into wedges
3 bacon strips, quartered and cooked until crisp

1. To make the dressing, in a small bowl, combine the olive oil, orange juice, orange zest, and chives, and season with salt and pepper. Set aside.

2. In a large salad bowl, combine the spinach and tofu. Add the dressing and toss until evenly coated.

3. Mound the salad on individual plates or on a platter. Top with the tomato wedges, egg wedges, and bacon.

4. Serve immediately.

The FODMAP Solution

Caesar Salad

Moderate FODMAP

Garlic-infused oil makes all the difference in this salad, since it delivers the punch of garlic without the galactans that could punch you in the gut. (See the recipe for Garlic-Infused Oil on page 60.) Use this salad as the foundation for a summer dinner, and fill it in with some grilled chicken, fish, or seafood.

4 tablespoons Garlic-Infused Oil (page 60)
2 tablespoons fresh lemon juice
1 teaspoon mustard
2 anchovy fillets (optional)
Kosher salt and freshly ground black pepper
6 cups chopped or torn romaine
3 tablespoons grated Parmesan cheese, plus more for serving
8 ounces cooked sliced chicken or shrimp (optional)
½ cup gluten-free croutons

1. To make the dressing, in a large salad bowl, combine the garlic-infused oil, lemon juice, mustard, and anchovies (if using), and season with salt and pepper.

2. Add the romaine and Parmesan. Toss until evenly coated and then mound on individual plates or a platter.

3. Top with chicken or shrimp (if using) and croutons. Serve immediately, with more Parmesan for sprinkling.

Niçoise Salad

Moderate FODMAP

A classic niçoise salad calls for canned tuna, but if you prefer grilled fresh tuna, use that instead.

4 tablespoons olive oil
2 tablespoons red wine vinegar
½ teaspoon mustard
2 tablespoons minced fresh chives
1 teaspoon dried oregano
Kosher salt and freshly ground black pepper

6 cups mixed salad greens
One 4-ounce can oil-packed tuna, drained
2 small tomatoes, cut into wedges
2 hard-cooked eggs, cut into wedges
1 cup fresh green beans, lighted steamed and chilled
4 small red potatoes, cooked, chilled, and sliced

1. To make the dressing, in a small bowl, combine the olive oil, vinegar, mustard, chives, and oregano, and season with salt and pepper. Whisk until evenly blended.

2. In a large salad bowl, combine the greens and half of the dressing. Toss until evenly coated. Mound the lettuce on individual plates or a platter.

3. On the top, arrange the tuna, tomatoes, eggs, green beans, and potatoes. Spoon the remaining dressing over the salad. Serve immediately.

Mediterranean Salad

Moderate FODMAP

There is some disagreement about exactly where peppers and chilis fall on the list of recommended foods for a low-FODMAP diet. Some lists exclude them, others include them. This recipe does not call for a significant amount of the peppers, but it is fine to leave them out. The salad has so many wonderful flavors and colors, you might not miss them.

¼ cup olive oil
2 tablespoons fresh lemon juice
1 teaspoon minced fresh mint
1 teaspoon minced fresh oregano
¼ teaspoon red pepper flakes (optional)
Kosher salt and freshly ground black pepper

4 cups chopped romaine lettuce
2 fresh tomatoes, cut into wedges
½ cucumber, cut into thin slices
10 Kalamata olives, pitted
4 anchovy fillets (optional)
¼ roasted red bell pepper, peeled and cut into strips (about ¼ cup)
2 teaspoons brine-packed capers, rinsed
2 teaspoons pine nuts
2 ounces cubed aged Provolone cheese
2 ounces cubed salami

1. To make the dressing, in a small bowl, combine the olive oil, lemon juice, mint, oregano, and red pepper flakes (if using), and season with salt and pepper. Set aside.

2. In a large salad bowl, combine the romaine, tomatoes, cucumber, olives, anchovies (if using), bell pepper, capers, pine nuts, Provolone, and salami. Add the dressing and toss until evenly coated.

3. Serve immediately.

81

Soups, Salads, and Sandwiches

Sloppy Joes

Moderate FODMAP

Molasses and coffee give these Sloppy Joes their flavor without any ketchup.

1 tablespoon olive oil
1 pound lean ground beef
1 tablespoon chili powder
1 tablespoon molasses
3 tablespoons coffee
¾ cup crushed tomatoes
4 gluten-free English muffins, toasted

1. Heat the olive oil in a large skillet over medium-high heat. Add the beef. Sauté, stirring frequently, until the meat is browned, 8 to 10 minutes.

2. Add the chili powder, molasses, and coffee. Stir well. Reduce the heat to medium-low and bring to a simmer. Stir in the tomatoes. Simmer until thickened and flavorful, 10 to 12 minutes.

3. Serve immediately on the toasted English muffins.

Tuna Melts

Moderate FODMAP

This recipe keeps the quantity of FODMAPs within suggested ranges, but if you find that the rye bread is a problem for you for other reasons, substitute another gluten-free bread or use the flatbread recipe in the previous chapter (page 63).

One 4-ounce can tuna, drained
3 tablespoons mayonnaise
2 tablespoons green onion, sliced (green part)
1 teaspoon minced fresh dill or ½ teaspoon dried dill
1 teaspoon fresh lemon juice
8 slices rye bread (wheat-free, gluten-free)
4 slices Swiss or Cheddar cheese
Butter, as needed

1. In a medium bowl, combine the tuna, mayonnaise, green onion, dill, and lemon juice. Stir together until evenly blended.

2. Divide the tuna salad evenly among 4 slices of bread. Top with the cheese. Add a second piece of bread to close each sandwich. Brush the outside of the sandwich with butter.

3. Heat a large cast-iron skillet or griddle over medium-high heat. Place the buttered sandwiches in the pan. Toast on the first side until golden brown, 4 to 5 minutes. Flip the tuna melts over, and toast on the second side until golden brown and the cheese is melted, an additional 3 to 4 minutes. Add a press to the sandwiches as they toast, for a crisper texture.

4. Slice in half. Serve immediately.

Panini

Moderate FODMAP

Mozzarella is a fresh cheese with far less lactose than whole milk. In fact, 30 grams of mozzarella contains less than 1 gram of lactose.

4 pieces Flatbreads for Pizza (page 63) or other gluten-free flatbread
8 ounces mozzarella, sliced and drained
8 tomato slices
½ teaspoon minced fresh thyme
½ teaspoon minced fresh basil
Kosher salt and freshly ground black pepper
1 tablespoon olive oil, or as needed for panini press

1. On each flatbread, layer the mozzarella, tomato, thyme, and basil, and season with salt and pepper. Fold the flatbread in half.

2. Heat a large cast-iron skillet or griddle over medium-high heat. Brush lightly with olive oil.

3. Add the panini. Griddle on the first side until golden brown, 2 to 3 minutes. Flip the panini over, and sear until the second side is golden brown and the cheese is melted, an additional 2 to 3 minutes. Add a press to the sandwiches as they toast, for a crisper texture.

4. Slice in half. Serve immediately.

Turkey and Brie Sandwiches

Moderate FODMAP

Avocados are considered moderate FODMAP food, so it is important to eat no more than the recommended serving size. This sandwich is a great place to include a few thin slices, as long as you can tolerate them.

8 teaspoons Sun-Dried Tomato "Hummus" (page 59)
4 pieces Flatbreads for Pizza (page 63) or other gluten-free
    flatbread, halved
12 ounces turkey slices
6 ounces Brie, sliced
4 avocado slices (optional)
4 tomato slices
2 cups gently packed fresh baby spinach
Kosher salt and freshly ground black pepper

1. Spread half the Sun-Dried Tomato "Hummus" on 4 pieces of flatbread.

2. Divide the turkey evenly among the 4 pieces of flatbread. Top with the Brie, avocado (if using), tomato, and spinach. Season with salt and pepper.

3. Spread the remaining hummus on the remaining 4 pieces of flatbread. Use those 4 pieces to close each sandwich.

4. Slice sandwiches in half. Serve immediately.

85

Soups, Salads, and Sandwiches

Reuben Sandwiches

Moderate FODMAP

Meats of all sorts are fine on the FODMAP diet, but preserved meats like corned beef, bacon, or sausages can include FODMAPs because of the way they are processed. Look for gluten- and lactose-free varieties. You can also find nitrate-free varieties from some specialty purveyors.

Cabbage is not a low-FODMAP food, because of the high amounts of galactans it contains. So here it is replaced with sliced dill pickle for some of the briny, savory taste of the more traditional sauerkraut.

4 teaspoons Dijon mustard
8 slices bread (wheat-free, gluten-free)
12 ounces sliced corned beef
2 dill pickles, thinly sliced
4 slices Swiss cheese
Kosher salt and freshly ground black pepper
2 tablespoons butter, room temperature

1. Spread half of the mustard on 4 slices of bread. Top with the corned beef divided evenly among the slices. Top with the pickle slices and Swiss cheese.

2. Spread the remaining mustard on the remaining 4 bread slices. Season with salt and pepper. Close each sandwich with the second slice of bread. Spread the butter on the outside of the sandwich to coat lightly.

3. Heat a large cast-iron skillet or griddle over medium-high heat. Place the buttered sandwiches in the pan. Toast on the first side until golden brown, 4 to 5 minutes. Flip the Reubens over, and toast on the second side until golden brown and the cheese is melted, an additional 3 to 4 minutes. Add a press to the sandwiches as they toast, for a crisper texture.

4. Slice in half. Serve immediately.

Appetizers and Sides

Note: Recipes in boldface are suitable for the first stage of the FODMAP diet. Recipes in regular type contain an ingredient that is a moderate FODMAP. Avoid eating these dishes within 3 hours of eating any other moderate FODMAP food, and limit portions.

Appetizers and Sides

Making a meal into an occasion calls for something out of the ordinary. Well-chosen appetizers and side dishes make the most of the main event. In addition to the recipes in this chapter, there are some other simple appetizer ideas to consider serving as a first course:

- steamed, grilled, or broiled seafood
- broiled grapefruit, sprinkled with a few grains of sugar
- marinated or pickled vegetables
- smoked fish (salmon, trout, whitefish)

Some simple side dishes can highlight the season and fill up your plate:

- steamed fresh green beans or corn
- leafy greens dressed with oil, lemon, salt, and pepper
- roasted vegetables

In addition to the suitable vegetables (page 20), you can also consider some moderate-FODMAP options, as long as you stay within the limits for the day.

Baked Brie with Cranberry Compote

Moderate FODMAP

The idea behind baking Brie is to give its already luscious texture a little boost so it is easy to spread and enjoy on gluten-free crackers or flatbreads. Or serve a wedge of baked Brie on a bed of greens with the compote for a beautiful and elegant first course to begin the meal, or a savory course to draw it to an end.

One 16-ounce bag fresh cranberries, picked over
½ cup orange juice
1 teaspoon grated orange zest
3 tablespoons maple syrup
One 12-ounce wheel or wedge Brie cheese (rind still on)

1. Preheat the oven to 350°F.

2. To make the cranberry compote, in a saucepan over medium heat, combine the cranberries, orange juice, orange zest, and maple syrup. Bring to a simmer. Cook, stirring frequently, until thickened, 8 to 10 minutes. Remove from the heat and let cool. The compote can be prepared in advance. Store in a covered container in the refrigerator for up to 4 days.

3. Put the Brie in a baking-serving dish and bake until the cheese is very hot, 12 to 15 minutes.

4. Serve at once, directly from the baking dish, accompanied with the cranberry compote.

Appetizers and Sides

Spinach Soufflé

MAKES 4 SERVINGS

Moderate FODMAP

Soufflés have a reputation for being finicky, which is true for classic soufflés made with a milk-and-flour base. In this version, however, the spinach adds body and the beaten whites make it rise. Will they fall when they come out of the oven? Yes, they will, so try to have everyone at the table when you are ready to serve.

Use the soufflé mixture to fill Buckwheat Crêpes (page 41) for an elegant appetizer.

Butter, at room temperature, for the soufflé molds
3 tablespoons Parmesan cheese, plus more for dusting
6 eggs, yolks and whites separated, at room temperature
12 ounces fresh or frozen spinach, cooked or thawed,
     squeezed dry, and chopped
Pinch of freshly grated nutmeg
Kosher salt and freshly ground black pepper

1. Preheat the oven to 400°F. Coat four 8-ounce soufflé molds with butter and dust lightly with Parmesan cheese. Set aside on a baking sheet.

2. In a large bowl, combine the egg yolks, spinach, 3 tablespoons of the Parmesan cheese, and the nutmeg, and season with salt and pepper.

3. In a large mixing bowl, beat the egg whites to medium-stiff peaks.

4. Fold the egg whites gently into the spinach mixture in three separate additions.

5. Spoon the batter into the prepared soufflé molds. Bake the soufflés on the baking sheet until they have risen and are lightly browned on top, 18 to 20 minutes.

6. Serve immediately.

Shrimp and Pineapple Skewers

MAKES 8 SKEWERS; 4 SERVINGS

First Stage FODMAP

As the pineapple broils, it adds a sweet-tart taste that stands in for a sauce. Use scallops or bite-size pieces of tuna or mahimahi, if you prefer. Turn this into a main course by serving the skewers on a bed of steamed rice.

1 pound extra-large shrimp, peeled and deveined
24 bite-size pieces pineapple
24 bite-size pieces red or green bell pepper
24 cherry tomatoes
8 bamboo skewers, soaked in water for 30 minutes
¼ cup olive oil
3 tablespoons fresh lemon juice
2 tablespoons minced fresh parsley
1 tablespoon minced fresh mint

1. Preheat the broiler to high. Adjust an oven rack so that it is about 3 inches from the heat.

2. Thread the shrimp, pineapple, bell peppers, and tomatoes divided evenly on the 8 skewers. Place the kebabs on the broiler pan.

3. In a small bowl, combine the olive oil, lemon juice, parsley, and mint and brush the kebabs generously with the marinade.

4. Broil, turning as necessary to cook evenly, brushing with marinade every few minutes, until browned and cooked through, about 12 minutes.

5. Serve immediately.

Turkey and Walnut Meatballs

First Stage FODMAP

These meatballs are tender and juicy, but if you want to serve a sauce or dip with them, try the Sun-Dried Tomato "Hummus" (page 59). Make these meatballs a little larger and simmer them in Tomato Sauce (page 122) to serve over your favorite gluten-free pasta for dinner.

1½ pounds lean ground turkey
1 egg, lightly beaten
1 cup finely chopped walnuts
½ cup minced green onions (green part only)
Kosher salt and freshly ground black pepper
2 tablespoons olive oil

1. In a large bowl, combine the turkey, egg, walnuts, and green onions, and season with salt and pepper. Mix with a wooden spoon or clean hands until evenly blended. Shape into meatballs about the size of marshmallows.

2. Heat the olive oil in a large cast-iron skillet over medium-high heat. Add the meatballs in a single layer. Cook, turning as necessary to brown evenly, until cooked through, 13 to 14 minutes. Transfer to a heated platter.

3. Serve immediately.

Beef Satay

First Stage FODMAP

A traditional satay includes peanut butter, but this recipe replaces the peanut butter with almond butter. Chiles are moderately high in FODMAPs, but a little goes a long way, especially if you choose something like a Thai bird chili. This recipe does contain soy sauce; however, many sources consider soy sauce, as well as tofu, suitable in limited quantities.

2 tablespoons molasses
3 tablespoons almond butter
2 tablespoons soy sauce
2 tablespoons thinly sliced chiles
2 tablespoons green onions, thinly sliced (green part only)
1 tablespoon ginger
1 tablespoon sesame oil
1 pound lean boneless beef (sirloin, tenderloin, or tri-tip),
    cut into strips
8 bamboo skewers, soaked in water for 30 minutes

1. To make the marinade and dipping sauce, in a small bowl, combine the molasses, almond butter, soy sauce, chiles, green onions, ginger, and sesame oil.

2. Put the beef strips in a 1-gallon ziplock bag. Pour half of the marinade over the beef, and reserve the other half to serve as dipping sauce. Turn to coat the meat evenly in the marinade. Marinate in the refrigerator at least 4 hours and up to 24 hours before grilling or broiling.

3. Preheat a grill or broiler to high. Remove the beef from the marinade. Thread on the 8 skewers.

4. Grill or broil, turning as necessary to brown evenly, until the beef is the desired doneness, about 6 minutes for medium-rare.

5. Serve at once, accompanied with the reserved dipping sauce.

Appetizers and Sides

Sautéed Swiss Chard

First Stage FODMAP

If you miss garlic, be sure to use Garlic-Infused Oil (page 60) for this brilliantly colored vegetable dish. See the note at the end of the recipe for details on how to prepare Swiss or ruby chard for this dish, as well as suitable alternatives to try.

2 tablespoons olive oil or Garlic-Infused Oil (page 60)
1½ pounds Swiss or ruby chard, separated into stems
    and leaves, chopped
½ cup chicken or vegetable broth
Kosher salt and freshly ground black pepper

1. Heat the olive oil in a cast-iron skillet or sauté pan over medium-high heat. Add the chard stems. Sauté until hot, 2 to 3 minutes.

2. Add the chard leaves. Sauté, stirring frequently, until the leaves are wilted, 5 to 6 minutes.

3. Add the broth and continue to cook until the stems are tender, another 3 to 4 minutes. Season with salt and pepper. Serve immediately.

The FODMAP Solution

Note: To prepare Swiss or ruby chard for a sauté, cut the stems from the leaves. Slice the stems into pieces about ½ inch long; keep the stems separate from the leaves, since they should go into the pan first. They need a bit more cooking time than the leaves. To cut the chard leaves, or other leafy greens, into ribbons, stack several leaves and then roll them into a cylinder. Cut crosswise to make strips.

Glazed Parsnips

MAKES 4 SERVINGS

First Stage FODMAP

Parsnips are delicately flavored with a natural sweetness. This dish presents them in a whole new light. The glaze comes from the addition of a little broth as the parsnips cook. A final addition of fresh parsley does more than make the dish look nice it adds a hint of flavor, as well as some important vitamins.

1 pound parsnips, peeled and cut into 1-inch pieces
½ cup chicken or vegetable broth
2 teaspoons fresh lemon juice
2 tablespoons butter
Kosher salt and freshly ground black pepper
2 tablespoons minced fresh flat-leaf parsley

1. In a shallow saucepan, combine the parsnips, broth, and lemon juice. Bring to a simmer over low heat. Cook, covered, until the parsnips are tender, 10 to 12 minutes.

2. Remove the cover and continue to cook, stirring occasionally, until all the liquid in the pan has evaporated.

3. Add the butter. Turn the parsnips in the butter until they are evenly coated.

4. Season with salt and pepper, and sprinkle with the parsley. Serve immediately.

Appetizers and Sides

Polenta

First Stage FODMAP

When polenta is served directly from the pot, it is soft and creamy like a porridge. The final addition of butter and cheese is optional, of course, but it makes the dish incredibly satisfying. If you have leftover polenta and put it in a dish to cool, it becomes firm enough to slice or cut into shapes. See the note at the end of this recipe for serving suggestions.

6 cups water
2 teaspoons sea salt, plus more for seasoning
¾ cup coarse yellow cornmeal (polenta)
3 tablespoons butter (optional)
¼ cup grated Parmesan cheese (optional)

1. In a large heavy saucepot, bring the water to a rolling boil over high heat. Add the salt.

2. Gradually add the polenta, a few tablespoons at a time at first, gradually increasing to a thin stream, and stirring constantly with a wooden spoon until thickened and pulling away from the sides of the pot, 25 to 30 minutes. Remove the pot from the heat. Stir in the butter (if using) and Parmesan (if using).

3. Season with additional salt if necessary. Serve immediately.

Note: Pour the polenta into a shallow baking dish or pie plate while it is still warm. Cool in the refrigerator until firm. Cut into wedges or slices, and then for an easy appetizer, panfry in olive oil or butter, broil, grill, or bake topped with sausage and tomato sauce.

Green Rice

First Stage FODMAP

This rice is cooked by the pilaf method, which will work for a number of other grains.

1 tablespoon olive oil
1 cup thinly sliced green onions (green part only)
1 cup long-grain basmati rice
1¾ cups chicken or vegetable broth
¼ cup minced fresh herbs, including one or more of the following:
    parsley, thyme, oregano, tarragon, basil, cilantro, chives
Kosher salt and freshly ground black pepper

1. In a saucepot over medium-high heat, heat the olive oil. Add the green onions and sauté, stirring frequently, until the green onions are vibrant in color, 1 to 2 minutes.

2. Add the rice and sauté until the rice is coated and smells toasty, about 2 minutes.

3. Add the broth. Reduce the heat to low and simmer the rice, covered, until the rice is tender to the bite, 15 to 20 minutes.

4. Fold in the herbs. Season with salt and pepper. Serve immediately.

Appetizers and Sides

Scalloped Potatoes

Moderate FODMAP

This recipe is a splurge dish, but is still low-FODMAP. Known in French as pommes Savoyard, *the addition of a nutty Emmental or Gruyère cheese makes this dish decadent.*

2 tablespoons butter, cubed, plus more for the baking dish
4 large russet potatoes, peeled and very thinly sliced
Kosher salt and freshly ground black pepper
1½ cups chicken or vegetable broth
2 eggs, lightly beaten
1 cup shredded Emmental or Gruyère cheese

1. Preheat the oven to 325°F. Coat a 1-quart casserole dish with butter.

2. Layer the sliced potatoes in the casserole dish. Season each layer with salt and pepper, and dot with the butter.

3. In a medium bowl, combine the broth and the eggs together. Pour over the potatoes. Sprinkle with the cheese. Cover with aluminum foil.

4. Bake until the potatoes are tender, 75 to 80 minutes. Remove the foil and continue to bake until the cheese is golden brown and bubbly, an additional 10 to 12 minutes. Let the scalloped potatoes rest a few minutes before serving.

Main Dishes

Crispy Tarragon Chicken

Chicken Curry

Chicken Saltimbocca

Jambalaya

Turkey Kefti

Navarin-Style Leg of Lamb

Pork Tenderloin with
Mustard-Horseradish Crust

Pork and Eggplant Stir-Fry

**Pan-Seared Flatiron Steak
with Tapenade**

Pot au Feu

Asian-Style Roast Beef

Meatloaf

Chili con Carne

Baked Spaghetti and Meatballs

Oat-Crusted Cod

Lemon Parsley Stuffed Trout

Cedar-Planked Salmon

**Caramelized Scallops with
Parsley Sauce**

Shrimp Diavolo

Vegetable Biryani

Tomato Sauce

Note: Recipes in boldface are suitable for the first stage of the FODMAP diet. Recipes in regular type contain an ingredient that is a moderate FODMAP. Avoid eating these dishes within 3 hours of eating any other moderate FODMAP food, and limit portions.

Main Dishes

Main dishes made predominantly from meats, poultry, fish, and seafood are generally safe on a low-FODMAP diet, as long as there are no inappropriate sauces or stuffings. If you are feeling like something special, you can always treat yourself to something luxurious, like scallops or shrimp, which are on the plan. Instead of a sirloin steak, splurge on tenderloin. If you miss the comfort foods you love, like meatloaf and fried chicken, you'll find recipes here.

Pasta is a popular entrée throughout the world, and it is good to know that there are low-FODMAP-friendly alternatives to wheat-based pasta. Quinoa, amaranth, rice, and corn are all used to make an array of noodles. Asian noodles are sometimes made from ingredients like sweet potato, buckwheat, and yam; check to be sure that the ingredients are on the list of suitable foods.

A few options in this chapter are good choices for "cooking ahead," leaving you with components for future meals. Some are great to make in a large batch and save in the freezer or refrigerator.

Crispy Tarragon Chicken

MAKES 4 SERVINGS

First Stage FODMAP

Tarragon is a classic combination with poultry, and in this dish, it is paired with a bit of mustard to mimic the flavor of classic fried chicken without the buttermilk or the deep-frying.

3 cups crumbled corn flakes (no sugar added)
3 tablespoons grated Parmesan cheese
1 teaspoon dried tarragon
Kosher salt and freshly ground black pepper
8 boneless skinless chicken pieces (thighs or breasts)
2 tablespoons mustard (optional)

1. Preheat the oven to 350°F. Set a rack in an ovenproof baking dish.

2. In a shallow dish, combine the cornflakes, Parmesan, and tarragon, and season with salt and pepper. Stir to combine.

3. Brush the chicken pieces with the mustard (if using) and then dredge in the cornflake mixture. Transfer to the rack in the baking dish.

4. Bake the chicken until it is golden and crispy on the outside and fully cooked (an internal temperature of 165°F), about 30 minutes.

5. Serve immediately.

Main Dishes

Chicken Curry

Moderate FODMAP

Curry pastes are sold in various colors to indicate their heat, from mild to fiery hot. Some are red, some yellow, some green, and some brown. Check the ingredient list carefully to be sure there are no FODMAPs in your favorite brand.

3 tablespoons olive oil or Garlic-Infused Oil (page 60)
8 chicken thighs, skin on, bone in
Kosher salt and freshly ground black pepper
One 2-inch piece fresh peeled ginger, chopped
1 large red bell pepper, chopped
3 tablespoons mild curry paste
1 tablespoon garam masala
1 tablespoon ground coriander
1 teaspoon ground turmeric
1 tablespoon dried fenugreek leaves
1 small red chili, thinly sliced
1 can coconut milk
½ bunch fresh cilantro, chopped
1 tablespoon chopped fresh chives

1. In a wide saucepot over medium heat, heat the olive oil. Season the chicken with salt and pepper, and sear in the hot oil on both sides, about 6 minutes total. Transfer to a plate.

2. Add the ginger, bell pepper, curry paste, garam masala, coriander, turmeric, fenugreek, and chili. Sauté, stirring frequently, until the bell pepper is tender, about 3 minutes. Add the coconut milk and bring to a simmer. Return the chicken thighs and any juices they may have released.

3. Simmer over low heat until the chicken is fully cooked, 15 to 20 minutes. Just before serving, stir in the cilantro and chives.

4. Serve immediately.

Chicken Saltimbocca

MAKES 4 SERVINGS

Moderate FODMAP

Saltimbocca is an Italian dish typically made with veal cutlets, but here, the veal is replaced with chicken. The word saltimbocca *means "jump in the mouth" because it takes no time at all once the chicken goes into the pan before it is ready to eat.*

4 boneless chicken breasts
4 thin slices prosciutto
12 fresh sage leaves
1 tablespoon olive oil
Kosher salt and freshly ground black pepper
2 tablespoons butter
Juice of 1 lemon

1. Butterfly the chicken breasts by making a horizontal cut almost all the way through the breast. Open it out and pound lightly to an even flatness.

2. Lay a piece of prosciutto on top of each chicken breast, and top with a sage leaf. Fold the chicken in half, enclosing the sage leaves. (There will be some sage leaves left.)

3. In a sauté pan over medium-high heat, heat the olive oil. Season the chicken with salt and pepper. Sauté in the hot oil until golden on both sides and cooked through, turning as necessary, about 15 minutes. Transfer the chicken to a platter or individual serving plates.

4. Return the pan to the heat. Add the butter, and when it stops foaming, add the remaining sage leaves. Cook until the leaves are crisp, about 2 minutes. Add the lemon juice and swirl to incorporate it into the butter. Pour over the chicken and serve immediately.

Main Dishes

Jambalaya

MAKES 4 SERVINGS

Moderate FODMAP

Rice-based dishes like this jambalaya are a great way to make filling and satisfying meals for yourself and your family. The usual chopped garlic is replaced with Garlic-Infused Oil (page 60) in this recipe.

1 tablespoon olive oil

2 skinless chicken breasts, diced

2 teaspoons Garlic-Infused Oil (page 60)

1 red bell pepper, thinly sliced

1 tablespoon chopped fresh chives

2 ounces Spanish-style chorizo sausage, sliced

1 tablespoon Cajun seasoning (check the nutrition label
    to make sure it's FODMAP-friendly)

1 cup long-grain rice

One 14-ounce can whole plum tomatoes, seeded and chopped

1 cup chicken or vegetable broth

1. Preheat the oven to 350°F.

2. In a Dutch oven or ovenproof and flameproof casserole dish, heat the olive oil. Add the chicken and sear on all sides until browned, about 4 minutes. Transfer to a plate.

3. Add the Garlic-Infused Oil, bell pepper, chives, chorizo, Cajun seasoning, and rice. Stir to coat the ingredients evenly. Add the tomatoes and broth and stir to combine. Return the chicken pieces. Cover and transfer to the oven. Bake until the rice is fully cooked, 20 to 25 minutes.

4. Serve immediately.

Turkey Kefti

First Stage FODMAP

A dipping sauce with yogurt or tahini is a nice addition to this dish. Choose a lactose-free or nondairy soy yogurt to avoid all FODMAPs.

1 pound lean ground turkey
1 tablespoon chopped fresh chives
1 tablespoon Garlic-Infused Oil (page 60)
1 teaspoon ground coriander
1 teaspoon ground cumin
2 tablespoons chopped fresh cilantro
Kosher salt and freshly ground black pepper
2 tablespoons olive oil as needed for shaping the kefti
8 bamboo skewers, soaked in water for 30 minutes

1. In a medium bowl, combine the ground turkey, chives, Garlic-Infused Oil, coriander, cumin, cilantro, and season with salt and pepper. Mix with a wooden spoon or clean hands until evenly blended.

2. Coat your hands with a little oil as you work to keep the turkey from sticking to your hands. Divide the turkey mixture into 8 equal portions. Shape 1 of the turkey portions into an oval. Press the skewer into the turkey, leaving one end to use as a handle. Squeeze the turkey around the stick and smooth the surface.

3. Heat the grill or a broiler to medium-high. Grill or broil the kefti, turning to brown and cook evenly, until cooked through, 12 to 13 minutes.

4. Serve immediately.

Navarin-Style Leg of Lamb

MAKES 4 SERVINGS

First Stage FODMAP

Navarin is a French stew of lamb or mutton. Let the lamb cook until it is just the doneness you like, but most chefs agree that a tender roast with a healthy blush of pink has the best flavor and texture. Choose fingerling, purple, or Russian banana potatoes for a special look and great flavor.

3 tablespoons olive oil
Juice of 1 lemon
1 tablespoon dried oregano
Kosher salt and freshly ground black pepper
One 3-pound boneless leg of lamb
6 Yukon Gold potatoes, peeled, cut into thirds
1 bunch baby carrots, trimmed

1. Preheat the oven to 350°F. Place a rack in a roasting pan.

2. In a small bowl, combine the olive oil, lemon juice, oregano, and season with salt and pepper. Brush the lamb with this mixture. Place the lamb on the rack in the roasting pan. Scatter the potatoes and carrots around the lamb and drizzle with a little of the olive oil mixture. Cover with foil and roast for 20 minutes.

3. Remove the foil, baste with the olive oil mixture, and continue to roast until the vegetables are tender and the lamb is cooked to the desired doneness, about 1 hour for medium-rare. An instant-read thermometer should register an internal temperature 135°F for medium-rare.

4. Let the lamb rest for 15 minutes before carving into slices. Serve on heated plates with the roasted vegetables. Spoon any pan juices over the lamb and vegetables.

Pork Tenderloin with Mustard-Horseradish Crust

MAKES 8 SERVINGS

Moderate FODMAP

Pork tenderloins cook quickly. They take less than half an hour to prepare, making this dish a perfect choice for busy nights, but they are elegant enough for a dinner party, too. This recipe can also be prepared on the grill, if you wish.

2 pork tenderloins, 5 to 6 pounds total
Sea salt and freshly ground black pepper

Mustard-Horseradish Crust
⅓ cup whole-grain mustard
2 tablespoons olive oil
2 tablespoons prepared horseradish, drained
1 teaspoon balsamic vinegar
2 tablespoons fresh thyme leaves
2 tablespoons fresh rosemary, finely chopped

1 cup chicken or vegetable broth
3 tablespoons butter

1. Preheat the oven to 375°F. Set a roasting rack in a roasting pan.

2. Trim the tenderloins to remove any fat or silver skin, if any, and season with salt and pepper.

3. In a small bowl, combine the mustard, olive oil, horseradish, vinegar, thyme, and rosemary. Rub the mixture all over the pork.

4. Transfer the pork to the rack in the roasting pan. Roast until a meat thermometer inserted in a roast registers an internal temperature of 145°F, about 20 minutes. Remove and let the pork rest for about 8 minutes before slicing and serving.

5. While the roast is resting, make a pan sauce. In the roasting pan, stir in the broth. Scrape any brown bits off the bottom of the pan and mix well to dissolve any drippings. Swirl in the butter and strain into a heated gravy boat or pitcher.

6. Serve the sliced tenderloin accompanied with the pan sauce.

Pork and Eggplant Stir-Fry

Moderate FODMAP

Bok choy is on the suitable vegetable list, but it is still a good idea to watch how much of it you have at a single sitting, since it is a type of cabbage.

Stir-Fry Sauce
1 cup chicken or vegetable broth
2 tablespoons chili paste (available from Asian grocers)
1 tablespoon rice vinegar
1 teaspoon toasted sesame oil
1 tablespoon cornstarch

¼ cup olive oil
1 pound ground pork
1 eggplant, halved lengthwise and cut into ½-inch-thick slices
1 tablespoon minced peeled fresh ginger
1 small red chili, finely chopped
2 heads baby bok choy, cut lengthwise into quarters

1. To make the stir-fry sauce: In a bowl, stir together the broth, chili paste, rice vinegar, sesame oil, and cornstarch. Set aside. Stir the sauce just before adding it to the stir-fry if the cornstarch has settled to the bottom.

2. Heat half of the olive oil, in a wok or skillet over medium-high heat. Add the ground pork and cook, stirring to break up any clumps, until it is thoroughly cooked, about 8 minutes. Transfer to a plate.

3. Add the remaining olive oil and when it is very hot, add the eggplant slices, working in batches to avoid crowding the pan. When the first side is cooked and brown, about 4 minutes, turn the slices over and cook an additional 4 minutes. Transfer the cooked eggplant to the plate with the pork.

4. Add the ginger and chili to the wok, and stir once or twice. Return the pork and eggplant to the wok, and stir to combine. Add the stir-fry sauce and cook until the sauce is thickened, about 2 minutes. Continue to cook and stir until the pork and eggplant are warmed through, another 3 minutes.

5. Serve immediately.

Pan-Seared Flatiron Steak with Tapenade

MAKES 4 SERVINGS

First Stage FODMAP

The tapenade in this recipe makes a great topping for grilled or broiled fish, or try it as an addition to sautéed greens. You can make the tapenade in double or triple quantities to keep on hand in the refrigerator for an instant sauce or spread.

Tapenade
½ cup pitted Kalamata olives
1 teaspoon Garlic-Infused Oil (page 60)
2 anchovy fillets, drained
2 tablespoons capers, rinsed and drained
2 teaspoons fresh thyme leaves
2 tablespoons minced sun-dried tomatoes (oil-packed)
Juice of ½ lemon

Four 8-ounce lean flat iron steaks
Kosher salt and freshly ground black pepper
2 sprigs fresh thyme or rosemary leaves, roughly chopped
1 tablespoon olive oil

1. To make the tapenade: In a food processor, combine the olives, oil, anchovies, capers, thyme, sun-dried tomatoes, and lemon juice. Purée, pulsing frequently, just until a coarse paste forms. Transfer to a small bowl and reserve. (If the tapenade is made in advance, store it in a covered container in the refrigerator for up to 1 week.)

2. Season the steaks with salt, pepper, and thyme. Let the steaks sit at room temperature for 15 minutes before pan-searing.

continued ▶

3. Heat a large cast-iron skillet over high heat. Add the olive oil, and when the oil ripples and looks hazy, add the steaks. Work in batches or use two skillets to avoid crowding the pan. Cook the steaks without disturbing until the upper surface looks moist, about 3 minutes. Turn the steaks once and reduce the heat to medium. Continue to cook until the steaks are browned on the second side and cooked to the desired doneness, 3 to 4 minutes for rare, or 4 to 5 minutes for medium.

4. Transfer the steaks to heated plates or a platter. Return the skillet to the heat. Add the tapenade to quickly heat it up. Pour the tapenade over the steaks and serve immediately.

The FODMAP Solution

Pot au Feu

First Stage FODMAP

A true pot au feu *calls for oxtail, tongue, and other meats, but this simplified version still has plenty of flavor, made from just a beef roast and chicken thighs. The cooking time is long, but the dish requires little attention beyond keeping it at a low simmer. One of the main reasons to make a pot au feu is the delicious, flavorful broth you'll have left to use in other dishes and the leftover beef to slice for sandwiches.*

One 3-pound beef brisket
8 cups chicken or vegetable broth
Kosher salt and freshly ground black pepper
2 chicken thighs, boneless and skinless, cut into 2-inch pieces
2 carrots, peeled and diced
1 celery stalk, peeled and diced
1 parsnip, peeled and diced
1 turnip, peeled and diced
1 cup peeled and cubed butternut squash
2 fresh thyme sprigs
2 fresh flat-leaf parsley sprigs
1 dried bay leaf

Dijon mustard
Gherkins or cornichons

1. Place the beef in a deep saucepot or Dutch oven and add the broth. If necessary, add water until the beef is covered by about 1 inch. Season with salt and pepper. Place over low heat and bring to a simmer, skimming the surface as necessary while the beef cooks. Continue to simmer slowly until the meat is about halfway done, about 45 minutes.

2. Add the chicken, carrots, celery, parsnip, turnip, squash, and herbs. Simmer until the beef is fork-tender and the chicken and vegetables are fully cooked, an additional 40 to 50 minutes.

3. Remove the beef and carve it into slices.

4. To serve the pot au feu, place the sliced beef, chicken, and vegetables in heated soup plates. Ladle the hot broth over the meat and vegetables. Serve immediately accompanied by mustard and gherkins.

Asian-Style Roast Beef

MAKES 6 TO 8 SERVINGS

First Stage FODMAP

The glaze in this recipe would be good on chicken breasts or thighs, pork tenderloin or pork chops, or a roast duck, as well as the beef.

Glaze
5 tablespoons prepared sweet chili sauce
Grated zest of 1 large lime
3 lemongrass stalks, finely chopped
One 2-inch piece fresh ginger, peeled and finely chopped
2 tablespoons olive oil

One 3-pound boneless beef roast (sirloin, top round, tri-tip, or rib)
Kosher salt and freshly ground black pepper

1. Preheat the oven to 350°F. Put a rack in a roasting pan.

2. To make the glaze: In a small bowl, stir together the chili sauce, lime zest, lemongrass, ginger, and olive oil. Set aside.

3. Trim the roast and season it with salt and pepper. Place the roast on the rack and brush it with the glaze. Roast to the desired doneness, about 1 hour (an instant-read thermometer inserted into the meat registering 135°F for rare). Brush the roast every 15 minutes with the glaze as it cooks.

4. Let the roast rest for 15 minutes before carving into slices. Serve immediately.

Meatloaf

MAKES 4 SERVINGS

First Stage FODMAP

Most meatloaf recipes call for bread soaked in milk, but oats are a perfect replacement. They give the meatloaf substance and help hold it together so that it slices well. Plus, the oats are a great absorber of moisture.

Cooking spray
1½ pounds lean ground beef
1 pound ground pork sausage
1 cup rolled oats (gluten-free)
2 eggs, lightly beaten
½ teaspoon hot red pepper flakes
1 tablespoon chopped fresh chives
Kosher salt and freshly ground black pepper
½ cup tomato sauce

1. Preheat the oven to 350°F. Coat a loaf pan with cooking spray.

2. In a large bowl, combine the beef, sausage, oats, eggs, hot red pepper flakes, and chives, and season with salt and pepper. Mix with a wooden spoon or clean hands until evenly blended.

3. Pack the meat mixture into the loaf pan in a loaf shape with some air space around the sides. Spread the tomato sauce over the top.

4. Bake, uncovered, until cooked through and an instant-read thermometer inserted into the loaf registers 150°F, 60 to 75 minutes.

5. Let the meatloaf rest for 15 minutes before cutting it into slices and serve hot.

Chili con Carne

MAKES 4 SERVINGS

First Stage FODMAP

Steamed rice is a traditional accompaniment to chili, but try it on a bed of creamy Polenta (page 96).

2 tablespoons olive oil

1½ pounds lean ground beef

1 teaspoon Garlic-Infused Oil (optional, page 60)

1 carrot, peeled and finely chopped

1 celery stalk, peeled and finely chopped

2 jalapeño chiles, seeded and minced (optional)

1 red chili, seeded and minced (optional)

2 tablespoons chili powder

1 teaspoon paprika

One 14-ounce can diced tomatoes, with their juice

1. In a Dutch oven or oven-proof casserole dish, heat the oil over medium-high heat. Add the beef and cook, stirring to break up any clumps, until thoroughly cooked, about 8 minutes. Transfer to a plate.

2. Add the Garlic-Infused Oil (if using), carrot, celery, jalapeños, red chili, chili powder, and paprika. Sauté, stirring frequently, until the celery is tender and translucent, 3 to 4 minutes.

3. Return the beef and any juices on the plate to the pot and add the tomatoes. Reduce the heat to low and simmer, stirring occasionally, until the beef is very tender and the chili is flavorful and thickened, 45 to 50 minutes.

Baked Spaghetti and Meatballs

Moderate FODMAP

Some nonwheat pastas are firmer than others, but almost every kind responds well to this American version of Italian comfort food. Be sure to cook the pasta just until it is barely tender, because it will continue to cook in the oven as it bakes.

1 pound gluten-free spaghetti (rice, quinoa, amaranth, etc.)
Twelve 2-ounce Turkey and Walnut Meatballs (page 92)
3 cups Tomato Sauce (page 122)
¼ cup shredded mozzarella or grated Parmesan cheese (optional)

1. Preheat the oven to 350°F.

2. Bring a large pot of salted water to a rolling boil over high heat. Add the pasta and cook until almost tender, according to package instructions. Stir to separate the spaghetti strands. Drain well and transfer to a 2-quart baking dish.

3. Top the spaghetti with the meatballs and cover with the sauce. Add the cheese (if using). Cover with foil and bake until very hot, 20 to 25 minutes. Remove the foil and bake until the cheese is melted and golden brown, an additional 4 to 5 minutes.

4. Serve immediately.

Main Dishes

Oat-Crusted Cod

MAKES 4 SERVINGS

First Stage FODMAP

Use the topping for any fish you like, or as a stuffing for butterflied shrimp or split lobster tails.

2 cups rolled oats (gluten-free)
½ cup chopped fresh flat-leaf parsley
2 tablespoons grated lemon zest
3 tablespoons butter or olive oil
Four 6-ounce cod fillets
Lemon juice, as needed for seasoning
Kosher salt and freshly ground black pepper
Lemon wedges for garnish

1. Preheat the oven to 375°F. Place a rack in a baking dish.

2. To make the oat crust, in a food processor, grind the oats, parsley, lemon zest, and butter together until crumbly.

3. Season the fish with lemon juice, salt, and pepper. Divide the oat crust evenly among the fish pieces, pressing lightly into an even layer. Place the fish on the rack in the baking dish. Bake until the fish is fully cooked and the flesh separates easily into large flakes, about 14 minutes.

4. Serve immediately, accompanied with the lemon wedges.

Lemon Parsley-Stuffed Trout

MAKES 4 SERVINGS

Moderate FODMAP

Use this stuffing with coho salmon or a similar pan-dressed fish, or use it as a topping for broiled shrimp or lemon sole.

¼ cup minced fresh flat-leaf parsley
¼ cup unsalted butter
Juice and zest of 1 lemon
4 brook trout, pan-dressed, about 2 pounds total
⅓ cup oat flour
Kosher salt and freshly ground black pepper
16 thin slices lemon

1. Preheat the oven to 375°F. Put a rack in a baking dish.

2. In a small bowl, combine the parsley, butter, lemon juice, and lemon zest, and mash it together with a fork until evenly blended. Divide the lemon butter evenly among the trout, spreading it on the inside of each one.

3. In a shallow bowl, add the oat flour and season with salt and pepper. Close the trout and dredge the outsides of the fish in the oat flour, shaking off any excess. Transfer to the rack in the baking dish. Top each trout with 4 slices of lemon, overlapping them.

4. Bake until the fish is completely cooked, 20 to 25 minutes (an internal temperature of 145°F). Serve immediately.

Cedar-Planked Salmon

First Stage FODMAP

Although not traditional for a cedar-planked salmon dish, the Cranberry Compote on page 89 makes a great accompaniment to the fish. Or, feature this salmon on a bed of Caesar or Spinach Salad (pages 79 and 78).

1 cedar plank (approximately 8 by 12 inches)
1 tablespoon olive oil
3 tablespoons brown sugar
1 tablespoon paprika
1 teaspoon ground cumin
1 teaspoon salt
½ teaspoon freshly ground black pepper
Four 8-ounce skin-on salmon fillets, pin bones removed

1. Soak the cedar plank in cold water for at least 2 hours.

2. Preheat a grill to high or an oven to 450°F.

3. In a small bowl, combine the olive oil, sugar, paprika, cumin, salt, and pepper.

4. Place the salmon on the plank and brush with the olive oil mixture. Place over indirect heat on the grill and cook covered, or bake in the oven until the salmon is cooked through, 16 to 18 minutes, depending on the thickness of the fillets.

5. Serve immediately.

Caramelized Scallops with Parsley Sauce

MAKES 4 SERVINGS

First Stage FODMAP

The trick to getting a rich, brown color on the scallops is blotting them very dry before you put them in the pan. The pan should be quite hot, almost smoking, and you should only add a few scallops at a time to not overcrowd the pan.

2 tablespoons olive oil

16 large scallops, cleaned (1 to 1½ pounds total)

Kosher salt and freshly ground black pepper

2 tablespoons butter

3 tablespoons sliced blanched almonds

2 teaspoons fresh lemon juice

2 tablespoons chopped parsley

1. In a large sauté pan over medium-high heat, heat the oil until it is hazy and the surface ripples. Blot the scallops dry with paper towels, season lightly with salt and pepper, and add to the hot oil. Work in batches if necessary. Sear the scallops on the first side until deep brown, about 2 minutes. Turn once, and sear on the second side, about 2 more minutes. Transfer the scallops to a platter.

2. When all of the scallops have cooked, reduce the heat to medium. Add the butter and cook until the foaming has subsided, about 1 minute. Add the almonds and cook until golden, about 2 minutes. Add the lemon juice and parsley and swirl the pan to combine. Spoon this sauce over the scallops and serve immediately.

Main Dishes

Shrimp Diavolo

First Stage FODMAP

Most classic Italian seafood recipes quite pointedly avoid putting cheese and seafood in the same dish, but if you like a little Parmesan cheese on top of this, no one will know but you.

1 pound linguini or fettuccini, gluten-free
¼ cup olive oil
1 red chili, roughly chopped
1 large handful fresh basil leaves, roughly chopped, plus
    more leaves for garnish
1½ pounds jumbo or extra large shrimp, peeled and deveined
¼ cup white wine
1½ cups Tomato Sauce (page 122)
Kosher salt and freshly ground black pepper

1. Bring a large pot of salted water to a rolling boil over high heat. Add the pasta and stir to separate the strands. Cook until tender, according to package instructions. Drain well and keep warm.

2. In a large skillet, heat the olive oil. Add the chili and basil leaves and sauté for about 1 minute, stirring constantly. Add the shrimp and cook, turning as necessary, until they turn a bright pink color, about 3 minutes. Add the wine and simmer until the wine has evaporated, about 2 minutes. Add the tomato sauce and simmer until the shrimp are fully cooked, about 8 minutes.

3. Serve the shrimp with the tomato sauce on a bed of pasta in heated pasta plates. Top with a few leaves of basil.

Vegetable Biryani

First Stage FODMAP

A good biryani has an appealing, crisp crust on the top, bottom, and sides of the dish. You can use any vegetables you like in the filling, or add some chopped or shredded meats, fish, or poultry.

Butter or ghee for brushing casserole, plus more for drizzling
3 cups cooked basmati rice
1 small carrot, peeled and sliced ½ inch thick
1 medium potato, peeled and cut into cubes
1 sweet potato, peeled and cut into small cubes
1 zucchini, cut into cubes
¼ red bell pepper, diced
1 cup chopped green beans
½ cup diced tomatoes
½ teaspoon minced red chili
1 teaspoon garam masala
¼ teaspoon ground turmeric
½ teaspoon toasted cumin seeds

1. Preheat the oven to 350°F. Brush a 2-quart casserole dish with butter.

2. Layer the biryani as follows: half of the rice, the carrot, potato, sweet potato, zucchini, bell pepper, green beans, tomatoes, and chili. Sprinkle the garam masala and turmeric over the vegetables. Add the remaining rice, spreading it into an even layer.

3. Drizzle the top of the rice layer with additional butter. Cover with foil and bake until the vegetables are tender, 20 to 25 minutes. Remove the foil and continue to cook until the top layer is browned, another 5 to 10 minutes. Sprinkle with the cumin seeds.

4. Serve immediately.

Tomato Sauce

MAKES 3 CUPS

First Stage FODMAP

Add other spices and herbs to give this sauce a new flavor profile. A pinch of cinnamon gives it a Moroccan flavor, while red pepper flakes make it bold and spicy.

2 tablespoons olive oil
One 14-ounce can peeled tomatoes, seeded and crushed,
    with their juice
1 tablespoon Garlic-Infused Oil (page 60)
1 teaspoon sugar (optional)
Kosher salt and freshly ground black pepper
3 to 4 large basil leaves

1. In a saucepot, heat the oil over low heat. Add the tomatoes and their juice and drizzle with the Garlic-Infused Oil. Bring the mixture to a simmer and cook, stirring occasionally, until the sauce has reduced by half and has thickened, about 40 minutes.

2. Taste the sauce and season with sugar (if using), salt, and pepper. Tear the basil leaves into the sauce and simmer until flavorful, about 3 minutes. Mash the sauce with a potato masher for a chunky texture, or for a smoother texture, purée the sauce with an immersion blender or in a blender.

3. The sauce is ready to use. It may be kept in a covered container in the refrigerator for up to 3 days or in the freezer for up to 3 months.

The FODMAP Solution

Desserts

Note: Recipes in boldface are suitable for the first stage of the FODMAP diet. Recipes in regular type contain an ingredient that is a moderate FODMAP. Avoid eating these dishes within 3 hours of eating any other moderate FODMAP food, and limit portions.

Desserts

If you have completed the initial stage of your FODMAP diet and have identified the specific foods that are problems for you, you can now begin to branch out with a few special treats, like the desserts in this chapter. While they are not always FODMAP-free, they are low-FODMAP items, so as long as you can tolerate a specific food, like butter or cream, for instance, you can have them in controlled portions.

Simple desserts to enjoy—really just something to satisfy that longing after dinner—include the following:

- Frozen ripe bananas, puréed with a little lactose-free milk for a quick and satisfying smoothie

- Nuts and cheese

- Strawberries (add a splash of cognac and a small sprinkle of sugar to enjoy them Romanov-style)

- Tropical fruits, like bananas, pineapple, and star fruit

Baked desserts on the low-FODMAP diet generally call for some flour and thickener with which you are probably becoming more familiar. Both brown and white rice flour, tapioca flour, potato starch, arrowroot powder, cornstarch, and xanthan gum are pantry staples if you plan to do much baking. You can find more information about baking without wheat and rye by consulting the Resources, page 139.

Strawberry Rhubarb Cake

Moderate FODMAP

Baking with yogurt gives this cake a subtle tangy flavor and a smooth, rich crumb. If you don't have yogurt on hand, you can make this cake with soured lactose-free milk or nut milk by adding 2 teaspoons lemon juice to 1 cup of milk and letting it sit for about 10 minutes.

Cooking spray
½ cup sliced almonds
¼ cup shredded dry coconut (unsweetened)
¼ cup packed light brown sugar
1½ teaspoons ground cinnamon
1¼ cups rice flour
⅔ cup almond flour or almond meal
⅓ cup tapioca starch (or corn flour)
2 teaspoons baking powder
¾ cup unsalted butter, at room temperature
½ cup granulated sugar
4 eggs
1 cup plain yogurt (lactose-free)
12 ounces rhubarb, trimmed and sliced
8 ounces strawberries, hulled and sliced

1. Preheat the oven to 300°F. Coat a 9-inch round cake pan with cooking spray.

2. In a small bowl, combine the almonds, coconut, brown sugar, and cinnamon, and toss together until evenly blended. Set aside.

3. In a medium bowl, blend together the rice flour, almond flour, tapioca starch, and baking powder with a whisk to break up any lumps and distribute the baking powder evenly.

continued ▶

4. Using the paddle attachment of a stand mixer or a wooden spoon and a large mixing bowl, cream together the butter and granulated sugar until very light and fluffy, about 4 minutes.

5. Add the eggs to the butter-sugar mixture, one at a time, blending well and scraping the bowl between each addition.

6. Add the flour mixture to the butter mixture in thirds, alternating with the yogurt, and mix until smooth. Pour the batter into the cake pan and spread it in an even layer.

7. Top the batter with a layer of rhubarb and strawberries. Scatter the coconut and almond mixture evenly over the fruit. Bake until a toothpick inserted in the cake comes out clean, 30 to 35 minutes.

8. Let the cake cool in the pan on a wire rack for 20 minutes before unmolding onto the rack.

9. Serve the cake warm, room temperature, or chilled.

Lemon Poppy Seed Cake

Moderate FODMAP

This is a dense, moist cake with a brilliant lemon flavor. Poppy seeds add crunch and flavor in this classic combination.

Cooking spray

Soaking Glaze
¼ cup confectioners' sugar
1 teaspoon cornstarch
2 teaspoons fresh lemon juice
1½ teaspoons cold water
½ teaspoon grated lemon zest

1 cup rice flour
½ cup granulated sugar
2 tablespoons poppy seeds
2 teaspoons baking powder
½ teaspoon xanthan gum
¼ teaspoon salt
½ cup milk (lactose-free)
2 tablespoons canola oil
1 egg
1 teaspoon lemon extract
1 teaspoon grated lemon zest

127

Desserts

1. Preheat the oven to 325°F. Coat an 8-inch round cake pan with cooking spray.

2. To make the soaking glaze: In a small saucepan, combine the confectioners' sugar and cornstarch, and stir to break up any lumps. Add the lemon juice, water, and lemon zest. Bring to a simmer over low heat, just long enough to thicken the glaze. Set aside.

continued ▶

3. In a large bowl, blend the rice flour, granulated sugar, poppy seeds, baking powder, xanthan gum, and salt with a whisk to break up any lumps and distribute the baking powder evenly.

4. In a small bowl, combine the milk, canola oil, egg, lemon extract, and lemon zest, and whisk to combine. Add this mixture to the flour mixture and stir to make a smooth batter. Pour the batter into the cake pan and spread it in an even layer.

5. Bake until a toothpick inserted into the cake comes out clean, 30 to 35 minutes. Let the cake cool in the pan on a wire rack for 20 minutes before soaking and glazing.

6. Using a bamboo skewer, poke holes over the surface of the cake and then brush the cake with the soaking glaze. Repeat two to three times, letting the cake soak up the syrup for a few minutes between each addition.

7. Chill the cake for 2 to 3 hours before unmolding to slice and serve.

Almond Cake

Moderate FODMAP

Top this cake with your favorite fruit. FODMAP options include pineapple, mango, or a few fresh berries.

Cooking spray
4 eggs, separated, at room temperature
²/₃ cup sugar
2 cups almond flour
Fresh berries for serving (¼ cup per serving; optional)
Coconut cream or almond cream, whipped, for serving (optional)

1. Preheat the oven to 325°F. Coat a 9-inch round cake pan with cooking spray.

2. Using a stand mixer, whip the yolks until they are very thick and foamy, about 4 minutes. Gradually add half of the sugar, a few tablespoons at a time, and whisk until the foam is thick enough to mound when it drops from the whisk onto the rest of the batter. Fold in the almond flour until evenly incorporated.

3. In a clean bowl with clean beaters, beat the egg whites until soft peaks form. Add the remaining half of the sugar, a few tablespoons at a time, while whisking until the egg whites reach medium-stiff peaks.

4. Gently fold the egg whites into the yolk mixture in three separate additions. Spoon the batter into the prepared pan.

5. Bake until a toothpick inserted into the cake comes out clean, 30 to 35 minutes. Let the cake cool in the pan on a wire rack for 20 minutes before unmolding.

Desserts

Carrot Cake

Moderate FODMAP

Dense and moist, this carrot cake is a great option to take along when you attend a potluck celebration. If you don't have all the flours suggested, look for a wheat- and gluten-free flour blend at the store instead.

Cooking spray
1 cup white rice flour
¼ cup brown rice flour
¼ cup tapioca flour
¼ cup potato starch
1 teaspoon ground cinnamon
1 teaspoon baking powder
½ cup plus 2 tablespoons unsalted butter
⅔ cup packed light brown sugar
2 eggs
2 cups grated carrots

Icing
One 8-ounce package cream cheese (lactose-free),
    at room temperature
½ cup confectioners' sugar
2 tablespoons lemon juice

1. Preheat the oven to 350°F. Coat a 9-inch round cake pan with cooking spray.

2. In a medium bowl, blend the white rice flour, brown rice flour, tapioca flour, potato starch, cinnamon, and baking powder with a whisk to break up any lumps and distribute the baking powder evenly.

3. Using the paddle attachment of a stand mixer or a wooden spoon and a large mixing bowl, cream together the butter and brown sugar until very light and fluffy, about 4 minutes.

4. Add the eggs, one at a time, blending well and scraping the bowl between each addition. Add the carrots and blend well. Fold in the flour mixture.

5. Pour the batter into the prepared cake pan and spread in an even layer. Bake until a toothpick inserted in the cake comes out clean, 30 to 35 minutes.

6. Let the cake cool in the pan on a wire rack for 20 minutes before unmolding. Cool completely before icing.

7. To make the icing: Using the paddle attachment of a stand mixer or a hand held mixer, cream the cream cheese and sugar until very light and fluffy, about 4 minutes. Add the lemon juice and mix well, scraping down the bowl to blend evenly.

8. Spread the icing on the top of the cake. Cut into slices and serve.

Vanilla Bean Rice Pudding

First Stage FODMAP

If you like, you could add up to 6 tablespoons of dark or golden raisins or currants to this pudding along with the milk to plump it up and add a special sweetness.

¾ cup uncooked white rice
1½ cups water
1 cup milk (lactose-free), plus ½ cup
⅓ cup sugar
1 teaspoon vanilla extract
¼ teaspoon salt
1 egg, beaten
1 tablespoon butter

132

The FODMAP Solution

1. In a large saucepan, combine the rice and water and bring to a simmer over medium heat. Cook, covered, until the rice absorbs the water, 15 to 16 minutes. Add 1 cup of the milk, the sugar, vanilla, and salt. Reduce the heat to low and continue to simmer, stirring occasionally, until the milk is thickened and the rice is very tender, an additional 15 minutes.

2. In a small bowl, whisk together the remaining ½ cup milk with the egg. Add about 1 cup of the hot rice pudding mixture and stir to combine. Add this mixture to the saucepan with the rest of the pudding, stirring it in with a whisk. Simmer for about 3 minutes, stirring constantly to keep the pudding smooth.

3. Remove the pan from the heat and stir in the butter. Pour the pudding into a pudding dish or individual pudding cups. Let the pudding cool to room temperature, and then cover and chill in the refrigerator for at least 3 hours.

Pumpkin Cheesecake Pie

MAKES ONE 9-INCH PIE; 6 TO 8 SERVINGS

First Stage FODMAP

There is no reason to feel deprived, even at holiday dinners, with this simple-to-make pie. The crust is pressed into place, instead of rolled out.

Crust
1½ cups almond flour
⅓ cup sugar
1 teaspoon ground cinnamon
¼ teaspoon salt
6 tablespoons unsalted butter, at room temperature

Filling
Two 8-ounce packages cream cheese, lactose-free,
    at room temperature
2 eggs
½ cup pumpkin purée
⅓ cup maple syrup
½ teaspoon ground cinnamon
½ teaspoon vanilla extract
¼ teaspoon ground nutmeg
⅛ teaspoon ground cloves

1. Preheat the oven to 350°F.

2. To make the crust: In a food processor, combine the almond flour, sugar, cinnamon, and salt. Add the butter and pulse the machine on and off until the butter is cut into fine pieces and the mixture looks like a coarse meal.

3. Press the mixture into a 9-inch pie plate, making an even crust that lines the bottom and sides of the pan.

4. To make the filling: In a food processor, combine the cream cheese, eggs, pumpkin purée, maple syrup, cinnamon, vanilla, nutmeg, and cloves, and mix until very smooth and evenly blended.

5. Pour the filling into the crust. Bake until the filling is set, about 40 minutes. If the crust becomes brown too quickly, shield it with strips of aluminum foil.

6. Let the pie cool to room temperature before slicing and serving.

Peppered Pineapple with Molasses Caramel Sauce

First Stage FODMAP

A scoop of lactose-free ice cream or sherbet would be a great accompaniment to this luscious dessert, but it stands on its own as well. Try it made with brine-packed green peppercorns that have been drained and lightly mashed instead of the black peppercorns. If you are cooking on your grill, try this dessert cooked over charcoal instead of in a sauté pan for a barbecued flavor.

2 teaspoons freshly ground black peppercorns
4 slices pineapple, about ½ inch thick
2 tablespoons butter
3 tablespoons molasses
2 tablespoons orange juice

1. Sprinkle the peppercorns evenly over both sides of the pineapple slices.

2. In a skillet over medium-high heat, melt the butter. Add the pineapple slices and cook until the pineapple is browned, about 2 minutes. Turn and brown on the second side, an additional 2 minutes.

3. Transfer the pineapple slices to individual dessert plates. Reduce the heat under the skillet to medium. Add the molasses and orange juice, and bring to a simmer, stirring to release any drippings in the pan.

4. Spoon the sauce over the pineapple slices and serve immediately.

Lemon Tart

Moderate FODMAP

If you are cutting back on coffee to just one cup a day, as many plans suggest, consider saving it to enjoy with a slice of this tart, tangy, creamy dessert.

Crust
1½ cups almond flour
⅓ cup granulated sugar
1 teaspoon ground cinnamon
¼ teaspoon salt
6 tablespoons unsalted butter, at room temperature

Filling
5 eggs
½ cup granulated sugar
½ cup plus 2 tablespoons butter, melted and cooled to room temperature
½ cup fresh lemon juice
Grated zest of 2 lemons

1. Preheat the oven to 350°F.

2. To make the crust: In a food processor, combine the almond flour, granulated sugar, cinnamon, and salt. Pulse in the butter until it is cut into fine pieces and the mixture looks like coarse meal.

3. Press the mixture into a 9-inch tart pan with a removable bottom, making an even crust that lines the bottom and sides of the pan.

4. To make the filling: In a medium bowl, combine the eggs, granulated sugar, butter, lemon juice, and lemon zest until evenly blended. Pour into the crust. Bake until the filling is set and the crust is browned, 25 to 30 minutes.

5. Let the tart cool to room temperature before slicing and serving.

Orange Polenta Soufflé

MAKES 6 SOUFFLÉS

First Stage FODMAP

If you enjoy chocolate and can eat it without any problems, try dropping a piece of dark chocolate into each soufflé just before serving.

Butter, for the soufflé dishes, at room temperature
½ cup fine yellow cornmeal (polenta), plus more
    for the soufflé dishes
3 cups water
3 large strips orange zest
½ teaspoon sea salt
4 eggs, separated, at room temperature
¼ cup sugar
3 tablespoons Grand Marnier
1 teaspoon finely grated orange zest

1. Preheat the oven to 400°F. Brush six 8-ounce soufflé dishes with butter. Dust the soufflé dishes lightly with a little cornmeal and set on a rimmed baking sheet.

2. In a large heavy saucepot, bring the water to a rolling boil over high heat. Add the strips of orange zest and salt.

3. Gradually add the cornmeal, a few tablespoons at a time at first, gradually increasing to a thin stream, and stirring constantly with a wooden spoon until the potenta is thickened and easily pulls away from the sides of the pot, 25 to 30 minutes. Pour the polenta into a shallow bowl, and let it cool. Remove and discard the orange zest.

4. In a medium mixing bowl, beat the egg whites to soft peaks. Add the sugar, a few tablespoons at a time while mixing, until the egg whites reach medium-stiff peaks.

5. In a separate medium bowl, stir together the egg yolks, Grand Marnier, and grated orange zest. Fold into the polenta until smooth.

6. Fold the egg whites into the polenta in three separate additions. Spoon the soufflé mixture into the prepared molds.

7. Put the baking sheet with the soufflés into the oven. Add about ½ cup water to the baking sheet. This will create some steam while the soufflés bake. Bake the soufflés until they have risen and have a golden color on top, 14 to 15 minutes.

8. Serve immediately.

Resources

Low-FODMAP Foods and Diets

FODMAPs: Fermentable, Oligosaccharides, Disaccharides,
Monosaccharides And Polyols
http://www.kcl.ac.uk/medicine/research/divisions/dns/projects/fodmaps/
index.aspx

The Monash University Low-FODMAP Diet
http://www.med.monash.edu/cecs/gastro/fodmap/

Stanford Hospital and Clinics Digestive Health
http://stanfordhospital.org/digestivehealth

Irritable Bowel Syndrome (IBS)

Irritable Bowel Syndrome Self Help and Support Group
www.ibsgroup.org

Irritable Bowel Syndrome (IBS) Health Center
www.webmd.com/ibs

Mayo Clinic Irritable Bowel Syndrome
http://www.mayoclinic.org/diseases-conditions/irritable-bowel-
syndrome/basics/definition/con-20024578

National Digestive Diseases Information Clearinghouse (NDDIC)
http://digestive.niddk.nih.gov

GERD

The GERD Diet
http://www.mckinley.illinois.edu/handouts/gerd_diet.html

Healthy GERD Diet
http://www.webmd.com/heartburn-gerd/

Recipe Index

Index

meatballs, 92, 115
meatloaf, 113
medicines, FODMAPs in, 16
meditation benefits, 9–11
minestrone, 73
muffins, 48

N
nuts
    pecans, 53
    suitable, 24–25
    walnuts, 46–47, 53, 67, 92

O
oil, 60
osmotic compounds, 7

P
pantry-stocking tips, 23–27
pasta dishes, 115
peptic ulcers, 9–11
pies, 133
pizza, 63–64
plaque, 6
polenta, 96, 136–137
pork dishes, 107–108
potatoes, 51, 55, 75, 98
prosciutto, 103
pudding, 132
pumpkin, 53, 133

R
relaxation benefits, 9–11
resources, 139
rhubarb, 125–126
rice dishes, 97, 132
roast beef, 112

S
salads, 69–86
sandwiches, 69–86
satay, 93
scones, 46–47
seafood dishes. *See* fish and
    seafood dishes
side dishes, 87–98
simple carbohydrates, 6
skewers, 91
small meals, 9–11
smoking cessation, 9–11
smoothies, 39
snacks, 57–68
soluble fibers, 6
soufflés, 90, 136–137
soups, 69–86
soy products, 25–26
spinach, 51, 78, 90
steak, 109
stir-fry dish, 108
sugar alcohols, 5
sun-dried tomatoes, 59

sweeteners, 25
Swiss chard, 94

T
tapenade, 109
thickeners, 26
tips
    baking, 26–27
    dining out, 28–29
    pantry-stocking, 23–27
tomato sauces, 122
tomatoes, 59, 72
tortillas, 74
turkey dishes, 55, 85, 92, 105

U
ulcerative colitis, 9–11

V
vegetables
    to avoid, 21–22
    to limit, 21
    suitable, 20–21
    vegetable dishes, 48, 51, 55, 62,
        66, 71, 75, 98, 121, 130–131

W
waffles, 42
weight loss, 14

Z
zucchini, 59, 68

CPSIA information can be obtained
at www.ICGtesting.com
Printed in the USA
LVHW081856020322
712195LV00012B/524